HOSPITALS
AND HEALTH

Your Orthomolecular Guide
to a Shorter, Safer Hospital Stay

ABRAM HOFFER, M.D., PH.D.
ANDREW SAUL, PH.D.
STEVE HICKEY, PH.D.

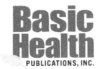

Basic
Health
PUBLICATIONS, INC.

The information contained in this book is based upon the research and personal and professional experiences of the authors. It is not intended as a substitute for consulting with your physician or other healthcare provider. Any attempt to diagnose and treat an illness should be done under the direction of a healthcare professional.

The publisher does not advocate the use of any particular healthcare protocol but believes the information in this book should be available to the public. The publisher and authors are not responsible for any adverse effects or consequences resulting from the use of the suggestions, preparations, or procedures discussed in this book. Should the reader have any questions concerning the appropriateness of any procedures or preparation mentioned, the authors and the publisher strongly suggest consulting a professional healthcare advisor.

Basic Health Publications, Inc.
www.basichealthpub.com

Library of Congress Cataloging-in-Publication Data

Hoffer, Abram
   Hospitals and health : your orthomolecular guide to a shorter, safer hospital stay / Abram Hoffer, Andrew Saul, Steve Hickey.

    p. cm.
   Includes bibliographical references and index.
   ISBN 978-1-59120-260-8 (Pbk.)
   ISBN 978-1-68162-734-2 (Hardcover)

   1. Hospital care—Popular works. 2. Patient education—Popular works.
I. Saul, Andrew W. II. Hickey, Steve III. Title.
   RA975.5.P38H64   2011
   362.11—dc22

                                    2010052423

Editor: John Anderson
Typesetting/Book design: Gary A. Rosenberg
Cover design: Mike Stromberg

Contents

Acknowledgments

After ninety-one years of a life very well lived, Dr. Abram Hoffer passed away while collaborating on this book. The co-authors continued with the project, editing and adding to Dr. Hoffer's text to generate what we hope is an accurate representation of his work. We cannot thank him enough for his humanitarianism, mentoring, and friendship. Few, if any, researchers or practicing physicians have had more influence on modern nutritional medicine than Abram Hoffer. Indeed, Linus Pauling himself first introduced the term "orthomolecular medicine" as a result of reading Dr. Hoffer's work. Our tribute to Dr. Hoffer is to publish this information.

We would like to thank the International Schizophrenia Foundation and its Executive Director Steven Carter for kind permission to use material that was first published in the *Journal of Orthomolecular Medicine*.

We would also like to thank Dr. Hilary Roberts for reading and making suggestions on an early version of the text.

Dangerous Places

"The doctor is often more to be feared than the disease."
—FRENCH PROVERB

Hospitals are dangerous places, and it is hard to find out whether or not they provide an overall benefit to society. Most people, over the course of their lives, are likely to spend some time in a hospital. What many may not realize is that the risks of becoming an in-patient can outweigh the benefits. Taken as a whole, a hospital's advantages might not outweigh the damage inflicted within.

Throughout history, hospitals have been places to stay away from. Entering a hospital meant you were more likely to die, whether from unnecessary infection or as a result of the treatment. Nowadays, we are told, advances in science and medical technology have changed this and hospitals are necessary and safe. Regrettably, this is far from accurate—hospitals can still be deadly.

Sometimes, of course, hospitalization is essential—in cases of severe trauma or other acute, life-threatening emergencies. Similarly, for complex, life-saving surgical procedures, with risks of complications, a well-equipped hospital may be vital. But, in general, they are to be avoided. Just as most people would think it irrational to enter an active war zone, so they should avoid hospitals—both are bad for your health. In high-tech societies, the over-commercialized and over-managed medical establishment is in serious trouble.

The harm done by corporate medicine and hospitals is enormous, but most people do not have a feel for large numbers or statistics. Think of this: in 1945, atomic bombs dropped at Hiroshima and Nagasaki killed approximately 200,000 people. Shockingly, each year, health care in the United States kills at least as many people as two atomic bombs dropped on large cities, the equivalent of a Hiroshima and a Nagasaki. This terrifying picture is not an overstatement: we are using recognized estimates of unnecessary medical deaths.

On entering a hospital as a patient, you endanger your health: there is a high risk of infection, complications, or even death. The reader might consider these statements unsupportable, biased, or alarmist. They are not. The risks associated with extreme sports, such as mountain climbing, swimming with sharks, or motor racing, can be lower than those of a hospital stay. As the United States begins to offer universal health coverage for its citizens, the risks of hospitalization will not magically go away. Indeed, more access means a higher likelihood of medically induced injury.

A DANGER TO YOUR HEALTH

It is generally assumed that, overall, hospitals are beneficial. This is speculation, however, as the risks to the patient if they avoid the hospital and remain untreated have not been quantified. One way of getting an idea is to measure what happens when doctors go on strike; in such cases, the death rate has been reported as declining.[1] In 2000, the *British Medical Journal* reported that when doctors in Israel went on strike, the death rates fell.[2] A similar fall in mortality was reported for a previous strike in 1983.[3] Death rate reductions have been reported during strikes in Israel (three separate occasions),[4] in Canada in the 1960s, and in England[5] and Los Angeles County in the 1970s.[6] The idea that hospitals are necessary and help the sick may be both obvious and quite wrong.

The effect of doctors' strikes may be considered an amusing anecdote in medical circles, but it is a finding that requires explanation. The most direct explanation is that medicine continues to be a leading cause of death. Modern medicine may at times provide useful treatments and save lives, but it is not clear that it provides an overall benefit. Medicine has inherent dangers. Those dangers are concentrated where there are the greatest numbers of practitioners, sick patients, and adventurous technologies. That place is a hospital.

The dangers of hospitals have been known for decades. In 1964, Dr. Elihu Shimmel published a classic paper documenting the finding that a patient entering hospital has a one in five chance of harm from an adverse event and a one in twenty-five risk of serious injury or death.[7] Since then, hospitals have continued to cause harm, which could be greatly reduced if simple controls were implemented.

The dangers associated with medicine, and hospitals in particular, are not controversial. A typical study, done by the Institute of Medicine, describes the risks of a stay in Boston's University Hospital.[8] These were defined as issues resulting from a diagnostic procedure or from any form of therapy. In addition, they included harmful occurrences (for example, falls or bedsores) that were not consequences of the patients' diseases. From a total of 815 consecutive patients, 36 percent suffered hospital-induced injuries; in 9 percent, injuries were considered severe enough to threaten life or serious disability. For fifteen patients, the hospital-induced illness "contributed to the death of the patient." In this study, patients entering the hospital had almost a one in fifty chance of dying from some cause other than their disease; if they had hospital-induced complications, the risk of death rose to one in twenty.

The Boston University Hospital study became the target of medical black humor[9] rather than a stimulus for change. However, the data suggest that the risk associated with a single hospital stay is greater than that of being killed in a motor vehicle accident over an entire lifetime (1 in 100).[10] In fact, the risk of suffering a fatal accident in a single hospital stay is similar to the lifetime risk of accidental death from any cause (one in thirty-six).

The Boston hospital was not singled out as being an accident black spot; rather, the risks reported are similar to those in other hospitals. The dangers of modern hospitals have been confirmed many times. If patients received optimal care, at least a quarter of hospital deaths might be avoided.[11]

Naturally, some doctors challenged these conclusions and suggested that the reports were exaggerated.[12] Firstly, they argued that the Institute of Medicine should not have compared hospital deaths to motor vehicle deaths, since hospitals were dealing with sick people, who are prone to die anyway. Also, the Institute's report dealt with only the sickest patients who would be expected to have a high death rate. They argued that the deaths were not necessarily caused by the hospital's errors; it could just have been that the people who died happened to have suffered the specified adverse events.

Harvard's Dr. Lucian Leape points out that the assumption that the patients concerned were the sickest group, who might have died anyway, is not valid. Many patients who died "were not very sick"; the hospital was responsible. Suggesting that doctors merely shortened the period of life is irrelevant—we all die eventually. Thousands of patients are dying, and hospitals are killing them. Leape's arguments are not easily dismissed. To suggest that the patients "would have died anyway" is scant consolation for relatives and is an unwarranted assumption.

In a study of 182 deaths from 12 hospitals, 14–27 percent of deaths from common causes, heart attack, pneumonia, or stroke were reported to be preventable.[13] These high mortality conditions accounted for over one in three hospital deaths.[14] Similarly, it was reported that 17 percent of intensive care patients had serious or fatal adverse events that need not have occurred.[15] In a study of 1,047 patients, 185 were reported to have had at least one serious adverse event. Patients who stayed longer in the hospital had more adverse events than those who where discharged quickly—the risk of an adverse event increased by about 6 percent for each day a patient stayed in the hospital. To compound this risk, about 18 percent of patients had serious events involving a longer hospital stay, increased costs, and increased risk of additional adverse events.

The number of unnecessary deaths in hospitals is alarming. About 2.5 million people die in the United States each year, and bad medicine may kill up to one in three of all people dying. These large numbers blunt the senses. Details of the death of a single child can tear at the heart, but 100,000 deaths is simply a statistic. Whether medical errors kill 44,000, 98,000, or 784,000 people each year in the U.S., as has been variously reported,[16] is not the point; even the least of these figures would be a glaring indictment of current medical practice. The lowest estimate places medicine firmly among the top ten causes of death in the U.S.; the highest makes medicine the number one killer.

MEDICAL PROGRESS?

A recent book by historian David Wootton concludes that, throughout most of its history, medicine has been harmful.[17] He argues that, over the millennia, medicine was generally unable to extend life and, for the most part, was detrimental to the patient. Around 1950, Wootton suggests, medicine became more scientific and patients benefited from greater health and longevity. This sounds reassuring, but would not a nineteenth-century physician have made similar claims about the eighteenth century?

Perhaps inevitably, an overly optimistic idea of medical progress has long been a core feature of the profession. This could reflect "the triumph of hope over experience," as Samuel Johnson remarked of a man who remarried following a previous unhappy marriage. More likely, doctors might find it hard to practice if they did not believe they were curing their patients more successfully than previous generations. Of course, modern doctors claim to be scientific—they would rightly be classified as quacks if they did not. Hindsight will show whether current practitioners are right or wrong. Nevertheless, 100,000 deaths or more per year from medical errors will be hard to live down.

We concede that medical technology has advanced, with organ transplants, body scanners, and many new drugs. However, this does not always mean that patients benefit: such innovations may do harm as well as good. An example of this Janus-faced aspect is the use of mammograms for breast cancer. Clearly, if screening finds a cancer that would have been fatal, allowing it to be removed, it is beneficial to that patient. However, if a patient is unlucky enough to get a "false positive" result, the mammography has wrongly identified something harmless as possibly being cancerous. This patient may undergo uncalled-for investigations, biopsies, or even surgery, radiotherapy, and chemotherapy, at a financial and emotional cost. In this case, they would have been better off without the screening. Such an example is not mere speculation: a Swedish team, publishing in *The Lancet,* found that "for every 1,000 women screened biennially throughout 12 years, one breast cancer death is avoided, whereas the total number of deaths is increased by six." In everyday language, the screening killed six times as many people as it saved. The benefits of modern medical technology are at best mixed.[18]

INSTITUTIONAL INCOMPETENCE

Medicine is entering the terminal phase of a disease that might be named institutional incompetence. Progression has been remarkably swift and is beyond anything one might have predicted. The problems assaulting medicine are caused by conflict of interest, poor management, and closed-minded professionals. The process is speeded by the drug industry, ineffective politicians, and lax government regulators.

Terminal illness is expensive, as desperate attempts are made to avoid the inevitable or, at least, to make the patient more comfortable. The illness affecting medicine is no exception. The costs of modern medical care systems are huge and rising. Insurance organizations, whether private or governmental, complain about the high cost of medical care, as they try to avoid paying for services. The National Health Service in the United Kingdom has grown to be the third largest employer in the world, after the Chinese Army and the Indian Rail Service.[19] It employs 1.3 million staff or about 2 percent of the U.K. population.

Similar problems have arisen with government health services elsewhere. An example is the plan developed in Saskatchewan, Canada, in 1950. The intent of Premier Tommy Douglas was to make medical care available to everyone, irrespective of their station in life, but the original framers did not foresee that such a worthy plan would become inadequate by the twenty-first century. During the following fifty years, a number of factors came into play, complicating medical care and increasing its costs. Food quality declined, resulting in poor nutrition and increasing chronic disease. Corporate medicine increased in size and importance, influencing medical teaching and practice. The popularity of drugs grew in parallel with corporate medicine's advertising budget. The ensuing dash for profit and patentability overrode old-fashioned notions of safety and clinical effectiveness, leading to increases in the number and prices of drugs. These factors have combined to increase the number of drug-related deaths; corporate medicine kills vastly more people than illegal drug pushers.

Fundamental Problems

There are fundamental problems with America's disease-care system. Here we list some of the issues:

- Financial conflicts of interest—Doctors, hospitals, and pharmacies make money when people are sick. The end result is care of the sick, with little preventive medicine. There is virtually no funding from mainstream medicine to support research into nutrition and prevention. For-profit companies cannot make money from cheap, nonprescription nutritional supplements that cannot be patented.

- Poor management—Hospitals are often not well run. For example, even basic measures to provide healthy nutrition to patients or prevent infections are not prioritized.

- Government out of touch with the people—Governments may change the way they fund our failing "health" systems, but the underlying problem continues on, fundamentally unchanged, with its drug-and-surgery orientation.

- Complacency and misinformation from health professionals—For decades, nutritionists and dietitians have argued that vitamin and mineral supplements are not needed if you just eat a balanced diet. It is a nice story, but it is only a story. They have no scientific support for such statements. Supplements are the only practical way that people can get 800 IU of good-quality vitamin E daily, the minimum amount that may help prevent most cardiovascular disease, the number one killer. Many people will need even more. Supplements are needed to get 3,000 mg or more of vitamin C daily, the minimum amount that is claimed to be reasonably protective against cancer. Vitamin D deficiency is rife, leading to winter epidemics of colds, flu, and more severe illness. Similarly, magnesium, calcium, and chromium deficiency is the rule, even in the U.S. Keeping cholesterol and saturated fat out of your diet will not help. Medicine has been based on such myths for too long.[20]

- Avoidance of individual responsibility for health—The elderly are the main users of the disease-care system and are the chief taxpayer-supported users. This age group is often resistant to diet and lifestyle change with less time to benefit than the young. What preventive health education the elderly are offered is as limited as the typical nursing home diet. People are treated for diseases but are not properly educated to maintain their health. Willing acceptance leaves many dependent on dispensary-style medical care. For a few cents a day, nutritional supplements might extend a person's life and well-being. The system has taught people to expect to be ill frequently, hold out their hand to receive a prescription, and go away.

"FIRST, DO NO HARM"

Hippocrates' famous axiom "First, do no harm" is often quoted by doctors and is included in some translations of the Hippocratic oath. It remains popular because of the continuing realization that, too often, doctors *do* cause harm. They injure their patients by simple errors, which include mistakes and miscommunication, poor prescribing, overdosing, and inappropriate surgery. The rule that a doctor should do no harm does not work when medical practice focuses on cutting into the human body or dosing it with chemicals that are dangerous enough to require prescription.

Hospitals are the cathedrals of modern medicine, yet they remain some of the most dangerous places on earth.[21] They provide a necessary and often lifesaving service for injuries and other traumas. However, do not assume that a hospital is necessarily a good place to have a medical emergency. Delays in defibrillation can lower the chances of survival from a heart attack. In hospitals, defibrillation may often be delayed.[22] Delayed defibrillation was associated with only about half the chance of survival (22.2 percent vs. 39.3 percent) compared with prompt treatment. Some have claimed that it is safer to have a heart attack in a casino or an airport than in a hospital, as help in the form of first aid and defibrillation might be provided more quickly.[23]

Hospitals are essential for treating the critically ill. For most people, however, hospital visits are unnecessary. If you want to remain healthy, stay away from hospitals, unless you have an urgent medical condition.

REAL HEALING

Hippocrates emphasized nutrition, exercise, and cleanliness for restoring good health—these were the basis of his medicine. In ancient days, there were few alternatives to using diet as therapy. Animals in the wild have no medical alternative. Humans now have advanced medical technologies, but that does not necessarily mean these new options are superior or safe. With most short illnesses, the body heals itself. A bandage does not repair damaged skin, it merely keeps the wound clean and in an environment that will aid healing. For many illnesses, the doctor needs to promote healing by stabilizing the patient and ensuring that food, warmth, and other needs are met. Hippocrates is remembered for his oath, but he also provided a large number of aphorisms to guide the physician. Many of these sayings refer to nutrition and healing[24]:

- "When the disease is at its height, it will then be necessary to use the most slender diet."

- "For extreme diseases, extreme methods of cure, as to restriction [of the diet], are most suitable."

- "Persons in good health quickly lose their strength by taking purgative medicines, or using bad food."

- "If one gives to a person in fever the same food which is given to a person in good health, what is strength to the one is disease to the other."

Modern medicine has forgotten that, in most cases, disease is self-limiting. The common cold is just one example. The doctor's interventions ideally help the body heal itself. This issue goes to the heart of the doctor-patient relationship. Provided the patient is not in a coma, the doctor-patient relationship is important. Patients may recover when treated by some doctors but not when given similar treatment by others with whom there is no therapeutic relationship.

Patients expect to be treated with respect, to be taken seriously, and to be healed, or at least that a serious attempt be made to help them heal. People often judge a doctor's worth on the old-fashioned doctor-patient relationship rather than technical knowledge or skill. This is surprisingly rational, as poor communication is a major source of medical error: if doctors are not listening carefully and actively, patients may not bring up important information. Care is also needed when doctors give information. For example, patients who do not understand discharge instructions are more likely to be readmitted to the hospital or end up in the emergency room.[25]

In medical schools, doctors are taught the importance of being scientific. In this context, "being scientific" means following the principles of evidence-based medicine, in which treatments must be "proven" by controlled clinical trial or by long established practice. This approach is increasingly imposed by the Colleges of Physicians and Surgeons. Medical colleges examine the technical capabilities of their members rather than how many of their patients get well. Practitioners are expected to conform to treatments recommended by the medical schools and are not encouraged to experiment with new (or old) ideas.

Unfortunately, many doctors are not trained in the scientific method. They think they are being scientific when they are simply repeating methods memorized in college or promoted by corporate medicine. They do not realize that genuine science is a trial-and-error approach or that authority is not science. Increasingly, doctors follow general "best practice" rules, which are aimed at a hypothetically average patient, or the current "standard of practice," which advocates conformity with other doctors. Patients, however, are individuals, so what helps one may not work for another.

Patients want their doctors to cure them or, if this is not possible, to relieve their symptoms. They do not care whether the treatment is scientific or not, only that it works. Doctors want to use "scientifically proven" methods, without realizing that science and proof are incompatible.[26] Thus, they use only those methods that the medical authorities and corporate medicine have assured them are scientific. This approach is safe (for the doctor)—doctors do not lose their licenses for being conventional.

If they became real healers—working for the benefit of patients—they would not care what method they used as long as their patients got better. They would also make strenuous efforts to do no harm. However, doctors following this approach run a serious risk of problems with the medical authorities, and few doctors risk their careers for the lives of their patients.

Time for a deep breath. You may feel that this has been a rather gloom-and-doom opening, but the thrust of this book is positive. It explains how to take back control and protect your health. Make sure you walk out of the hospital's front door and do not end up on a slab in the basement.

BE RISK AVERSE

This book is divided into two main sections:

- **Part One: Diagnosis—Hazardous to Your Health.** This section looks at the problems with modern corporate medicine and why it can make a stay in the hospital dangerous to your health.

- **Part Two: Antidote—Patient Power.** This section offers suggestions for taking charge of your own health care.

Because of the possible dangers of modern medical care, patients need to be risk averse. This book offers some suggestions for minimizing the risks of being in the hospital. These are a summary of the actions we would take if we could not avoid a hospital stay. However, it is important to tailor your approach to your own circumstances.

We have written this book as a general and informative guide, for individuals who wish to lower their risk of death or injury while in the hospital. We believe that people should think for themselves, taking control of decisions about their health. A typical, intelligent person can take full responsibility for such decisions. Clearly, it would be foolish not to take into account the advice of doctors, nurses, and other health professionals. Sometimes, however, people become subservient and relinquish their authority to the hospital. Then, when things go wrong, the patient blames the doctor, resulting in a litigious environment where everyone loses.

Some of our suggestions involve dietary changes or supplements as these are considered central to maintain good health. But in certain cases, supplements are contraindicated; often, this is because of interactions with drugs or treatments. For example, the drug warfarin prevents blood clotting by blocking the action of vitamin K; thus, a patient would be unwise to simultaneously take a vitamin K supplement, as it is the antidote to the drug. It is always important to check the contraindications and side effects of any drugs you are taking. Since some doctors display a knee-jerk opposition to supplements, ask for specific reasons why you should not take any particular nutrients.

This book's aim is to help people steer clear of unnecessary risks and, if hospital treatment is unavoidable, to help increase the chances of a successful outcome. Your life depends on you taking personal responsibility for your health.

. . . .

PART ONE

Diagnosis— Hazardous to Your Health

CHAPTER 1

How Did We Get Here?

"Who are the greatest deceivers? The doctors?
And the greatest fools? The patients?"
—Voltaire (François-Marie Arouet, 1694–1778)

Criticisms of modern medicine may sound new but, historically, have been rather consistent. A 1929 editorial by Dr. F. H. Garrison in the *Bulletin of the New York Academy of Medicine* is entitled "The Evil Spoken of Physicians and the Answer Thereto."[1] Dr. Garrison draws on similar work from the seventeenth century, itemizing what he calls "these rusty weapons and damp ammunition, formerly employed so continuously to belittle our profession." Dr. Garrison lists the accusations as follows:

- The doctor usually kills rather than cures.

- Nature, left to herself, will usually heal the patient, but drugging may harm or kill him.

- The doctor is a pompous, pedantic, ceremonious duffer, who talks learnedly out of books to conceal his ignorance of reality.

- In medical consultations, the patient is slain by the force majeure of numbers.

- The demands of professional ethics and etiquette were formerly such that it was deemed better for a patient to die by rule (secundum artem) than to recover in defiance of medical principles. This affectation of legality or pontifical infallibility is, and has been, the weak link (in the eyes of enemies) in medical practice. It is here naturally that the quack finds his opportunity and gets his innings.

- The doctor trades upon illness, gets rich through the prevalence of disease, whenever it does not affect himself or impoverish his clientele.

- He pours medicines, of which he knows little, into bodies of which he knows less.

Such criticisms have dogged medicine for centuries. To quote Dr. Garrison, "For over twenty-five centuries, at least, these stereotyped slurs were cast up against physicians without let or hindrance." In other words, denigration of the medical profession has been happening since before the days of Hippocrates (circa 460–370 BC) in ancient Greece.

Each generation of doctors tells us their equivalent of the claim that medicine has become more scientific, with technical advances and modern methods that are assumed to render it more effective. Although they admit that old-fashioned medicine was of slight benefit, or even blatantly harmful, successions of medical authors proclaim that their new methods will save more lives and make people healthier. Unfortunately, much of this optimism is self-serving balderdash. As time passes, the deficiencies of previous medical paradigms, such as bloodletting or leeches, become apparent. They are not, however, necessarily replaced by effective and efficient health care. In the future, it seems highly likely that many of the methods so valued by our current physicians will be recognized as obviously harmful, and people will wonder why we were so gullible.

Dr. Garrison supports the current medicine of his day, using a familiar sequence of arguments, which we have extracted here:

- Medicine [in 1929] has become scientific and effective.

- The harm done by earlier physicians was a result of them working in an age of relative ignorance.

- Modern medicine has great scientists working unselfishly for the common good.

- Modern doctors have higher ethical and professional standards.

- Doctors work themselves to near extinction looking after their patients' health.

- A doctor with a bad reputation will soon lose his clients.

- The criticisms of medicine are humorous and not to be taken seriously.

Dr. Garrison suggests that, by 1929, medicine had conquered infectious disease and had perfected surgery, gynecology, obstetrics, dentistry, and the new science of infant welfare. In 1850, he suggested, people in the United States had no health whatever, but by 1929 they were healthy and athletic. Implicit in this is the suggestion that medicine had triumphed over illness. There is some truth in the idea that people had become healthier. However, much of the progress arose through better sanitation, hygiene, and nutrition. Over the last century, medicine has often taken credit for these improvements, while hiding the harm it causes.

A HISTORY OF SHAME

Organized medicine has a long history. As long as 6,000 years ago, medical schools were attached to ancient Egyptian temples. Hippocrates seems to have believed his treatments could cure disease and increase life span, but he was probably wrong. Hippocratic medicine (emetics, cautery, purgatives, and bloodletting) appears to have killed more than it cured. While Hippocrates placed emphasis on diet and exercise, he did not report the central importance of diet to health and longevity.

Infirmaries have existed since before the days of the Romans.[2] Back then, gladiators were revered as valuable sources of entertainment, like modern sports heroes. Chief physician and surgeon to the gladiators was Galen (129–199 AD), who attempted to repair their injuries. He thus gained the opportunity to see aspects of human anatomy without engaging in the then illegal practice of dissecting dead bodies. However, scientific progress was slow and treatments were based on faith rather than rationality.

From the time of the Greeks and Romans through to the nineteenth century, medicine relied on the four humors theory. The four humors—black bile, yellow bile, phlegm, and blood—were thought to fundamentally control health. When these four humors were in balance, the person was healthy, whereas if a particular humor increased or decreased, it caused weakness and ill health. Today, we might find this funny (humorous), but for much of history it was a medical disaster. A doctor might think a patient had too much blood and would therefore bleed the sick person, weakening him and preventing recovery. By contrast, phlegmatic patients were prescribed wine to return them to balance, so were probably happier, if not healthier!

For centuries, Galen's influence dominated medicine. Indeed, despite its claims to a scientific basis, the profession has been dominated by belief in authorities for most of its history. Galen was revered almost as a deity and, until the Renaissance, his work was considered definitive. In the sixteenth century, a notable polymath named Paracelsus helped break this stultifying tradition. Paracelsus had little time for modesty or self-effacement—his adopted name means "as great as or greater than Celsus," the Roman physician who had been influential for over a millennium. The word *bombastic* is sometimes said to arise from Paracelsus' original name, Phillippus Aureolus Theophrastus Bombastus von Hohenheim. While this may be historically incorrect, it gives a clear impression of the man. As an indication of his contempt, Paracelsus reputedly burned the books of Avicenna and Galen at the medical school in Basle.

To its shame and the detriment of its patients, medicine has consistently followed authority rather than working rationally from reason and data.

Bloodletting and Cautery

It should come as little surprise to the reader that early treatments for disease could be worse than the malady itself. Cautery was often used for minor ailments and was treated by physicians as something approaching a panacea. An early treatment for piles was cautery, which means to burn away dead tissue. Naturally, many people would prefer hemorrhoids to the application of a red hot poker. Quite likely, the mention of the word would have persuaded any hypochondriacs that they had made a rapid recovery.

Bloodletting had a long history despite the clear harm that it caused. It seems quite astonishing that the practice could continue for centuries without doctors noticing the stream of dead patients. George Washington was killed largely by his doctors' overenthusiastic bloodletting. They took an estimated 3.75 liters of blood over a period of nine to ten hours in December 1799.[3] An average adult has a total of about 4.7 liters of blood in their body. Washington had a bad cold, a throat infection and a fever, so his doctors bled him to death. Today, with hindsight, we can recognize these eminent doctors as quacks.

The historical benefits of medicine can be gauged by the observation that, from the time of Hippocrates to the middle of the nineteenth century, bloodletting was a universal remedy. The *Merck Manual* was still recommended bloodletting for some ailments as late as the 1934 edition.

Galen also advocated bloodletting, alongside a proper diet. For most maladies, a doctor in the time of the Romans could have provided medicine about as effective as that given in the early nineteenth century.

Mesmer and the Quacks

Some quacks are so famous that their names have become generic. Franz Anton Mesmer (1734–1815) lived around the time of George Washington and the term *mesmerize* means to enthrall, spellbind, or otherwise put someone into a trance. While generally considered a quack, Mesmer may have been the first successful clinical hypnotherapist. He certainly made a name for himself, and a good living, from his specialist treatment of the diseases of the rich.

Though called a quack, Mesmer is not known to have killed anybody. It might be argued that he diverted people away from authorized medicine, and, in so doing, caused them harm. However, at the time he was working, conventional treatments included mercury, purging, bloodletting, leeches, and so on. Diverting patients from such treatments might well have been doing them a favor. In Mesmer's era, doctors did not even wash their hands between patients. They would go from lancing a boil to delivering a baby, and from dissecting a cadaver straight to the operating theater. When compared with the available medical technology, Mesmer and his methods might reasonably be preferred by rational patients.

George Bernard Shaw provided a clear and characteristically amusing description of the difference between quacks and qualified doctors: "The distinction between a quack doctor and a qualified one is mainly that only the qualified one is authorized to sign death certificates, for which both sorts seem to have about equal occasion." Notably, Shaw died at the age of ninety-four, from injuries sustained falling off a ladder while pruning an apple tree. Few doctors live that long, never mind retaining the ability to climb trees.

BIRTH OF THE HOSPITAL

One puzzle that spans the history of medicine is why people were willing to pay doctors for treatments that didn't work and often harmed. If patients paid for treatments only when they were cured, it might have been a powerful economic constraint, and the financial incentive could have driven medical science to develop effective treatments. Even more baffling is why this practice of paying for ineffective and harmful treatment is tolerated today.

The early centuries of medicine had one great advantage—the patient paid the doctor and maintained responsibility and control. Later, the state or other large organizations (such as an insurance company) paid the doctor; as a result, patients lost control over their own bodies and health. As payment from the patient became indirect, doctors took more control. This situation brings us to the birth of the medical organization, the clinic, and the hospital. Historically, hospitals have provided an administrative convenience that transferred power to the medical profession but offered few benefits to patients.

At first sight, hospitals seem to be an obvious development. They bring economies of scale, centralized teaching, and the beginnings of organized medicine. French philosopher Michel Foucault suggests that as hospitals developed, the experimental method started to be applied and staff began using laboratories for investigation.[4] However, Louis Pasteur (1822–1895), often called the "father of modern medicine" and one of the most famous French scientists, worked in a laboratory in his own house. Until recently, hospitals were not necessary for many of the major developments in medical science.

Hospitals have helped organize medical investigations. In the nineteenth century, physiology developed rapidly as a discipline, based on dissection of cadavers and live animal experiments (vivisection, often without benefit of anesthetic). In Australia, at least as recently as 1973, live marine toads were routinely vivisected for neuromuscular experiments in biology courses. In Dr. Saul's physiology classes, the laboratory went through bushel-baskets of toads (admittedly a national pest) each week.

Over time, medicine became a science based on laboratory experiments. New disciplines, such as pharmacology and medical bacteriology, arose to provide medicine with the core scientific data it needed. For the patient, however, modern hospitals brought a shift away from good health as the key objective. Rather than helping a patient to become and stay healthy, the idea became to return them to normalcy.

Hospitals brought new teaching methods and a change in the doctor-patient relationship. Early hospitals helped doctors rather than patients. When patients benefited, it was likely to have been through chance and serendipity. From the early days of teaching hospitals, it became clear that they harmed patients, and initial statistics showed that a hospital was not a healthy place in which to be sick. Four in ten amputations resulted in death, for example. Sir James Simpson (1811–1870), discoverer of chloroform anesthesia, stated that "A man laid on an operating table in one of our surgical hospitals is exposed to more chances of death than was the English soldier on the field of Waterloo." One problem was that infection rates in hospitals were high, primarily because many sick people were contained in the same unhygienic building, thus increasing the opportunity for contagion.

Perhaps we should remind ourselves that Pasteur, who contributed so greatly to medicine's understanding of infections and their treatment, was not a physician. In fact, Pasteur was reluctant to work with medical doctors because he found them untrustworthy and resistant to progress. In 1885, Pasteur tested his rabies vaccine on a nine-year-old boy, Joseph Meister, who had been bitten by a rabid dog. However, Pasteur did this at great risk to himself: since he was not a physician, he might have been prosecuted. The deciding factor was that, without the vaccine, the rabies would have killed the boy. Both Pasteur and the boy were saved by the vaccine's success.

While Pasteur ignored the rules, he still succeeded in introducing important developments. Other medical innovators have faced great difficulties. Ignaz Semmelweis (1818-1865) attempted to get doctors in obstetric clinics to wash their hands in order to prevent the spread of childbed fever. Apparently, his colleagues considered this an outrageous suggestion. Semmelweis ended his days in a mental hospital, after years of fighting the medical establishment. Historian David Wootton, author of *Bad Medicine,* puts the position clearly, "Once doctors decided they need pay no attention to microorganisms, they immediately ensured that they would never have to encounter evidence suggesting they had made the wrong choice."[5]

People have suggested that if Semmelweis had been more easygoing and cooperative, his ideas might have been accepted earlier.[6] The counter argument is that if Semmelweis' personality were different, the problem and solutions may not have occurred to him, and he might not have had the courage to stand up for his crusading ideas. Even if he had started out with a most affable personality, it is unlikely that he would have retained it under the pressures to which he was exposed.

The Hygiene Paradigm

Semmelweis rebelled against a widespread problem by fighting the medical establishment. Without a paradigm change, however, he was fighting a losing battle. In his day, the standard of medical hygiene was low, particularly in hospitals. The medical establishment would have needed to change their views on the importance of hygiene. In effect, they would have had to admit they had been killing their patients. Doctors would take some time to reach that conclusion.

History suggests that reason and data can be ignored for generations: social revolutions involve a paradigm shift and take time.[7] This delay is particularly the case with medicine. To be told, in effect, "your dirty hands are killing people" was too much for the doctors to accept, even though it was true. Instead, by making small advances over time, hygiene could be incorporated into normal practice without loss of face. Indeed, it could be used as a demonstration of medical advancement.

By the middle of the nineteenth century, hospitals were death traps and were consequently in the process of becoming obsolete. They were dirty and dangerous places, to be avoided at all costs. Florence Nightingale introduced improved hygiene standards, but keeping a hospital clean does not prevent all infections. Hospitals were saved by a fundamental change in medical science—the theory of germs. The germ theory of disease allowed workers to understand the need for hygiene, the basis for antiseptics, and, ultimately, the use of antibiotics. At first, antibiotics were viewed as so powerful that they would defeat infectious disease forever.

The idea that advancing medical technology might overcome infections completely displays both arrogance and a misunderstanding of biology. Single-celled organisms are everywhere and, in biological terms, medicine is largely irrelevant. Modern hospitals are still plagued by rampant infection despite, or sometimes because of, the use of antibiotics. Bacteria have the ability to become resistant to drugs; the more a drug is used, the more likely it is that resistant bacterial strains will develop.

Nowadays, overuse of antibiotics has resulted in multi-drug (or methicillin)-resistant *Staphylococcus aureus* (MRSA), vancomycin-resistant *Staphylococcus aureus* (VRSA), and multi-drug-resistant tuberculosis (MDR-TB). The early successes of hygiene and antibiotics led to a reasonable expectation that a patient should be safe from infection when in medical care. The reality is different—modern hospitals remain a major source of some of the most dangerous infections.

AN ALTERNATIVE MEDICAL HISTORY

Modern medicine originated largely in the West and benefited from the Renaissance, Industrial Revolution, and the consequent rapid increase in scientific knowledge. In other parts of the world, notably China and India, practitioners developed independent forms of medical understanding and techniques.

The Chinese system is derived from Tao, Buddhist, and Confucian philosophies. In this view, a person's health is in a close relationship with their food and environment. An example is the concept of *yin-yang* balance, which in some ways is similar to the four humors of early Western medicine. Chinese philosophy differs greatly from modern biology and medicine, which has no direct counterpart to the concept of life force, *qi*, or the meridian system that is used in acupuncture. Indeed, some regard *qi* as pseudoscience,[8] while others describe it as a valid philosophical construct. Some adherents of Western medicine have described traditional Chinese medicine as a pre-scientific discipline. This may reflect a drive to eliminate competition, as shops selling Chinese medicines are becoming commonplace in Western shopping malls.

Acupuncture derives from traditional Chinese medicine and is often considered an alternative treatment in the West. Since there was no known physiological mechanism to explain results obtained by sticking pins in apparently imaginary lines on the surface of the body, acupuncture was initially rejected as a treatment. This rejection was essentially scientific but rather strange, as the dominant Western paradigm of "evidence-based medicine" is founded on statistical association rather than direct causation. Despite the apparently irrational nature of acupuncture, it seems to work. Acupuncture has been found to help low back pain,[9] postoperative nausea,[10] nausea and vomiting induced by cancer chemotherapy,[11] headache,[12] and dental pain. The claimed benefits of acupuncture are too numerous to list here and the clinical trials are inconsistent.

Clinical research into alternative therapies can be difficult. Unlike a drug, it is difficult to find a suitable placebo control for acupuncture. The person is typically aware that someone is sticking needles or applying skin pressure. A similar problem occurs in studying conventional surgery, where an ethical placebo operation is difficult to design and implement. Fortunately, the seemingly surprising positive results in some clinical trials have guided researchers to study the mechanisms involved. We now have direct evidence of a physiological effect.

Acupuncture can reduce pain by increasing pain thresholds.[13] A small pain can induce feedback, causing the release of brain hormones, which block larger pain signals. These hormones are similar to morphine and codeine, in that they are blocked by the drug naloxone. Also, like opiate drugs, repeated acupuncture generates both tolerance and cross-tolerance with morphine. When compared with a placebo, acupuncture pain relief takes time to develop and is more lasting, as might be expected from the physiological mechanisms. However, it appears that all forms of acupuncture are not equally effective for providing analgesia. In particular, electro-acupuncture seems best at delivering stimuli to activate powerful opioid and non-opioid analgesic mechanisms. To evaluate the efficacy of acupuncture, we need carefully controlled clinical experiment, rather than the crude trials currently employed.

Ayurvedic medicine is a legacy of developments on the Indian subcontinent. It began 5,000 years ago, with a greater degree of organization being introduced from about 1,500 years BC. *Ayurveda* means "knowledge of life" or biology. Indian medicine has provided alternative medicine with techniques such as yoga, massage, and a range of herbs, in addition to dietary advice. Traditionally, Ayurvedic medicine describes the body as consisting of blood, bone, chyle (or plasma), fat, flesh, marrow, and reproductive tissue (e.g., semen). There are three "humors": *vata* (driving force, e.g., nervous energy), *pitta* (fire, e.g., metabolism), and *kapha* (water, e.g., plasma), which need to be balanced for health. Hinduism and Buddhism were influential in its historical development. Notably, hygiene is an essential and valued part of Ayurvedic medicine.

Ayurvedic medicine is a complete health-care system using diet, exercise, meditation, and herbs to maintain mental and emotional health. It would be wrong to assume that this form of alternative medicine is somehow primitive compared with the Western approach. For example, the *Sushutra Samhita,* a book from Sushruta, who is known as the father of Indian surgery and lived perhaps around 600 BC, describes remarkable advances. It describes ulcers as unclean and needing to be cleaned before fully healing. It mentions that wounds can be stitched to prevent bleeding, and numerous types of surgery are covered. With the passage of time, it is not clear how successful these surgical interventions were. However, at least in some cases, cataract surgery was successfully performed with specific instruments as far back as 1,000 BC.[14] Sushruta even described nose jobs (rhinoplasty). Today, Ayurvedic medicine is becoming increasingly scientific, as it adopts the experimental method and clinical trials.

One of the main objections to Ayurvedic medicine is that some of its herbs can contain high levels of heavy metals. Manufacturing control of such herbs may be poor and about one in five medicines sold on the Internet contains lead, mercury, or arsenic.[15] Monitoring of quality is important.[16] This contamination relates to inadequately controlled companies supplying herbs rather than being a problem with the principles of Ayurvedic medicine. It is important to be sure that herbs are obtained from reputable suppliers.

The benefits of Indian medicine can be outstanding. Turmeric, for example, is a powerful antioxidant,[17] anti-inflammatory,[18] neuroprotective,[19] and anticancer[20] agent. Modern medicine is only just coming to terms with the properties of turmeric and the curcumins it contains. There are numerous other Ayurvedic treatments that may take decades to evaluate properly. Orthodox medicine would do well to show a little humility before dismissing these treatments.

ORTHODOX VS. UNORTHODOX MEDICINE

By the mid-nineteenth century, we entered an age of free-market medicine. Prescribed medicines and patent remedies shared a common feature—many were poisonous. Then, a number of doctors rebelled against their own profession by recommending vegetarianism, fasting, water, sunlight, and even exercise to cure the many diseases of the day. One of these was James Caleb Jackson, M.D. (1811–1895), developer of the first whole-grain breakfast cereal ("granula," later to be known as granola). Similarly, John Harvey Kellogg, M.D., of Battle Creek Michigan, was well known as an advocate of natural, high-fiber foods. His brother, Will Keith Kellogg, invented wheat flakes and the even more popular cornflakes. These pioneers in nutritional medicine followed the Hippocratic rule, "First, do no harm."

Today, doctors are arguably the most powerful professional group in society. In a sense, you do not exist as a legal human being until a doctor autographs your birth certificate and you are not free from paying taxes until your death certificate is signed. Doctors enjoy high incomes, high social status, and immense authority. Dr. Robert Mendelsohn, author of *Confessions of a Medical Heretic,* likens them to modern day priests and medicine to a new religion. A fundamental difference between science and religion lies in their respective reactions to challenge. In science, challenging a hypothesis is a core part of the methodology; in religion, it is considered heresy. We are so used to thinking of medicine as a respected and benevolent force that suggestions such as "more people live off cancer than die from it" are hard to accept. Nonetheless, the view of modern medicine as a business, profiting from sickness and suffering, is rational and consistent with the facts.

Unorthodox medicine has always been a specific target for criticism by doctors. In any science, there is disagreement, which is essential to drive progress. To the extent that medicine ultimately gains its authority from science, it needs open dialog, covering all rational approaches. In the health professions, open discussion keeps practitioners aware that there are varied approaches to health. Problems arise when one school of treatment achieves political power and can bias laws, limiting alternative schools of treatment. The American Medical Association (AMA) has largely achieved this goal. Although it represents fewer than half the physicians in the United States, it remains a powerful lobby in Washington, D.C., and an influential union or guild. Such behavior is unscientific, but it is typical of both religions (stamping out heresy) and commercial businesses (destroying the competition).

There is only one scientific criterion for an effective therapy: either it works or it does not. However, clinical trials are often designed and run for the benefit of corporate medicine.[21] The effect of this is to deny funding to trials of cheap, non-patentable therapies that might be effective but could damage corporate profits. Such untested treatments will be described as "unproven" and be ignored.

Few people who understand the history of modern medicine can regard it with any degree of pride. For many years, even the suggestion of basic hygiene during surgery was rejected. Western medicine gained its dominance from its commercial success. In the West, the development of science substituted experiment and observation for belief in authorities such as Galen. It is arguable that recent developments (such as evidence-based medicine) have tended to reverse this trend and have instituted a new form of authority-based medicine.[22]

In the East, Chinese and Indian forms of medicine have had a long history, with philosophical similarities to some early Western developments. In some respects, they were more advanced. However, the introduction of experimental science and advances in technology provided an advantage to Western medicine. This was reinforced by the commercial advantage of patents. Many of the methods of Chinese and, especially, Indian medicine have yet to be tested in clinical trials. This does not mean they do not work—just that they are untested in the required type of statistical clinical trial.

Modern medicine has come to consist of those treatments that provide financial profits. Furthermore, evidence-based medicine can repress proper scientific consideration of alternatives.

CHAPTER 2

Corporate Medicine and the Profit Motive

"He that takes medicine and neglects diet
wastes the skills of the physician."

—Chinese Proverb

The United States alone spends over $2 trillion each year on disease care. Despite this huge expenditure, U.S. citizens are only number 37 in the ranking of world health. In total, about 1,300,000 Americans have died in all the wars in U.S. history, yet today the U.S. loses a similar number of Americans each year from cardiovascular disease and cancer. Many of these premature deaths are avoidable.

Total drug industry sales are approaching $500 billion per year, half of which are in North America. Profit margins are so high that in some recent years "the combined profits for the ten drug companies in the Fortune 500 were more than the profits for all the other 490 businesses put together."[1] Drug companies make profits from the sick and view the healthy as potential profit centers. Hospitals have become industrial centers for extracting money from the ill and infirm.

SICKNESS = PROFITS

The U.S. has recently passed landmark legislation expanding its health-care delivery system. Many other countries have a national health service and they are beset with the same fundamental problem: their purpose is not improving health but treating sickness.

Sickness is profitable. So much so that, throughout the history of medicine, there have been quacks, making money peddling treatments and "cures." There are vast profits to be made in pharmaceuticals, medical technology, and delivery. However, these profits depend on people being sick. A sick person is often both desperate and vulnerable. A terminal disease is literally and psychologically a matter of life and death, and people will grasp at straws in hopes of a cure. The response to this has been to introduce legislation controlling who can treat the sick and what therapies can be used. Unfortunately, this well-meaning approach has produced a monopoly for corporate medicine.

Preventive medicine does not have the heroic appeal of treatment. Life-and-death surgery is dramatic and its results are immediate. Taking a daily supplement is less glamorous and the effects of improved nutrition are subtle. A person may not realize they are aging more slowly for many decades. They simply did not need a heart bypass. Even in such cases, assigning the person's longevity and health to their nutrition is difficult. However, preventive medicine is far more important than treatment. If modern medicine were based on prevention and the engineering dictum "If it ain't broke, don't fix it," the need for corporate medical care would collapse. We would need fewer hospitals and the financial and other medical costs could be 10 to 100 times lower.

Consider the question of whether patients need to be in a hospital. Robert Mendelsohn, M.D., describes the time he decided to minimize the number of patients on his ward.[2] He thought that many patients were on the ward unnecessarily and their health might improve if they were properly treated at home. Dr. Mendelsohn was in charge of twenty-eight beds with, initially, twenty-four patients. Having control over admissions, he checked each new patient to make sure they really needed to stay in the hospital. He arranged taxis for outpatient visits and a truck for adjusting patients' equipment, such as leg traction. With time and vigilance, Dr. Mendelsohn reduced the number of occupied beds to three or four; the other two dozen beds were unoccupied.

However, Dr. Mendelsohn quickly found that his patients were more necessary than he was. The nurses started to complain that they had nothing to do and were worried about being transferred. The young doctors did not have enough material for their studies. Dr. Mendelsohn's experiment ended rather quickly, a result that, in hindsight, was predictable. Look at these problems from the viewpoint of each of the players in turn: the nurses and doctors need patients in order to have a job; medical students need them in order to learn; the hospital needs patients in order to exist. Thus, the only people gaining when patients avoided hospitalization were the patients themselves. However, the patients were passive and did not have a lot of influence. They obeyed their doctors' orders to have hospital treatment. A doctor who reduced the number of patients treated in a hospital can expect to quickly be moved on. Furthermore, this might happen even in government-run hospitals with waiting lists and targets. The medical system needs patients, even if treatment does not benefit them.

MEDICAL DISASTER

There is a critical branch in the path of health education, and it occurs at the point where the subject is nutrition. Traditional, mainstream dietetics favors a balanced, all-food-groups diet, and discourages the use of food supplements. However, a persistent minority of nutritionists favor radical diet revisions and the therapeutic use of high-dose vitamin preparations. Fortunately, people can make up their own minds.

Throughout our lives, we make many crucial, this-or-that decisions: whether or not to attend college, whether or not to marry, which job to accept or not accept, whether or not to have children, and so on. Collectively, our society makes proportionally major choices with each political and economic decision, and with each election.

Today, the United States is engaged in developing a national health-care delivery system that will apparently continue to avoid alternative healing methods. America's national health-care scheme, if it is implemented, is likely to replicate the costly mistakes other nations have already made. By 1993, just the single Canadian province of Ontario had run up an enormous $12 billion debt, largely due to nationalized health care.[3] Universal health coverage is not a panacea: it will cost plenty and produce little. A change in funding is not a change in content.

Making pharmaceuticals and treatments more widely available will not solve the disease problem any more than making guns available solves the crime problem. At least half of all illnesses are avoidable, being due to unhealthy lifestyles and eating habits.[4] Extending catastrophically poor health care does not prevent disease.

Our expensive and ineffective health care systems are fundamentally unworkable. Even the most creative of financial makeovers will not save them. Assigning responsibility for our health to someone else is a central issue with a long history.

PATENT MEDICINE

Medicine developed with the medieval guilds in Europe, which can be viewed as a forerunner of the corporation. In current terms, guilds were something between a trade union and a secret society. It has been suggested that guilds provided an infrastructure for innovation and development.[5] However, eventually the restriction of free trade they imposed was recognized and action was taken to limit their influence. Ironically, the modern patent system helped to break the power of the guilds. Technological secrets that were being held as the property of a guild were made public, in exchange for a government-supported monopoly.

Patent medicines developed in the 1600s, when Letters Patent were issued by royalty. These seals of approval were used in advertising, rather like the "By appointment to Her Majesty the Queen" labels used in the United Kingdom on favored products. The term *patent medicine* was later used to describe numerous remedies, and such medicines reached the height of their popularity in the late 1800s, competing with bloodletting and purgatives. They included willow bark and its later derivative, aspirin. Physicians' ineffective remedies struggled to compete with the aggressive advertising of the patent medicines.

In the twentieth century, regulations were introduced and the U.S. Food and Drug Administration (FDA) was formed. Patent medicines had a poor reputation. It might be thought that patent medicines would have been regulated out of existence, but they are the core of modern medicine. Aspirin was a patent medicine of Bayer, now the third largest pharmaceutical company in the world. Today, many mainstream pharmaceutics are protected by patent, providing a monopoly to the drug company. However, companies avoid the designation "patent medicine," which was a synonym for quackery.

BIG PHARMA

Leading medical journals regularly carry critical analyses of the role of corporate medicine in the deterioration of the practice of medicine. They are careful, as many leading medical journals are funded by the drug advertisements they contain. Meanwhile, other members of the medical profession go along with the industrialization of medicine because of its financial incentives. Some medical journals are trying to break away from biases forced on them by the financial might of the pharmaceutical industry.

Making Bad Food Legitimate

Dr. Harvey Washington Wiley was the first chief of the U.S. Bureau of Chemistry, the direct forerunner of the Food and Drug Administration (FDA). He helped bring about the Pure Food and Drug Act in the first decade of the twentieth century. Dr. Wiley oversaw research on food additives to see if they were harmful to health. In a now rare and out-of-print book, *A History of a Crime Against the Food Law* (1929), he described the need for, and the findings of, this research[6]: "The total number of substances studied was seven, namely, boric acid and borax, salicylic acid and salicylates, benzoic acid and benzoates, sulfur dioxide and sulfites, formaldehyde, sulfate of copper, and saltpeter (sodium nitrate). Reports of these investigations were published, with the exception of sulfate of copper and saltpeter, which were denied publication."

The question is why publication of facts relevant to people's health was denied. This denial was of concern because the findings were that these additives were definitely harmful to health. Dr. Wiley wrote, "Vigorous protests from those engaged in adulterating and misbranding foods were made to the Secretary of Agriculture against any further publicity in this direction. As a result of these protests, he (the Secretary of Agriculture) refused publication of Parts VI and VII of Bulletin 84. Part VI contained a study of the effects on health and digestion of sulfate of copper added to our foods. The conclusions drawn by the Bureau were adverse to its use. The seventh part treated the use of saltpeter, particularly in meats. Owing to the well-known results of the depressing effects of saltpeter on the gonads, and for other reasons, the Bureau refused to approve the use of this coloring agent in cured meats."

Oddly this opinion changed with time, because the FDA allows nitrates and nitrites in our food and particularly in meats. This change occurred despite accumulating evidence of harm from nitrates and nitrites in food. Dr. Wiley's interpretation of the Pure Food and Drug Act of 1906 was this: "Following the rule adopted by the Bureau, every doubtful problem was resolved in favor of the American consumer. This appears the only safe ethical ground to occupy. Decisions against the manufacturers who used these bodies (*sic*) could be reviewed in the courts when the food law became established, whereas if these doubtful problems had been resolved in favor of the manufacturers, the consumer would have had no redress."

> In other words, Dr. Wiley's policy was that if there was doubt that an additive was safe, it should not be in food. How things have changed. The FDA allows 60 insect fragments in 100 grams of chocolate, 150 fragments in cocoa powder, and 10 mg of mammalian excreta in a pound of cocoa beans.[7] All food is contaminated but most people are unaware of how much. While insect fragments are unappealing, some additives, such as monosodium glutamate (MSG), may destroy brain cells and cause chronic disease.[8]

Former editors of the *New England Journal of Medicine,* for example, have published books about the pernicious effect of the drug companies on modern medicine.[9] These books add to a growing library documenting the malign influence of what has become known as "Big Pharma."[10]

Many people are worried about drugs, especially after reading about those such as Vioxx (rofecoxib), a painkiller that was voluntarily withdrawn by Merck in 2004 after being implicated in thousands of heart attacks and strokes. No wonder some patients tear up prescriptions as soon as they leave the doctor's office. Andre Picard recently reported that about $100 million worth of drugs in Canada are disposed off, usually by flushing them down the toilet.[11] Drugs have joined pesticides as an important source of water pollution.[12] Many years ago, cynics against nutritional supplements criticized vitamin C supplements, claiming incorrectly that only the fishes benefit. We are waiting for these guardians of our waters to comment about these drugs, which damage not only the fish but also humans who drink the water and eat the fish. Modern sewage systems are not good at removing the hormones, drugs, and chemicals that we dispose of in this way.

Corporate medicine's main concern is to sell their drugs for profit. They do this using modern techniques of advertising, sending representatives (drug reps) to doctors, and inviting doctors to support their drugs.[13] This process has extended to the point where drug companies write research papers, reviews, and speeches and then pay doctors for putting their names on them. Unwitting or not, too many doctors are working for corporate medicine rather than for their patients. We do not wish to dwell on this influence as, unless a person is particularly naive or uninformed, they will understand the problem of people who profit from the sick.

UNACCEPTABLE RISK

A patient entering a good hospital has about a one in twenty-five chance of suffering an adverse event.[14] Recently, the Healthcare Commission in the United Kingdom accused a "flagship hospital" in Staffordshire, England, of causing the deaths of hundreds of patients.[15] Appalling emergency care resulted in "enormous suffering." The limitations of this hospital were publicly highlighted. Unfortunately, the numbers of hospital deaths occurring each year suggest that even good hospitals are losing many patients to unnecessary death and suffering. Shortly after the problems at Staffordshire were disclosed, Basildon and Thurrock University Hospitals were found to be contributing to 400 deaths a year through filthy wards, poor nursing, and bad management.[16] Surprisingly, the Care Quality Commission, a government organization to validate hospitals, classified these hospitals as "good," giving them a score of 13 out of 14 for safety and cleanliness, and "excellent" for management. The hospital trust reportedly has a budget of about $400 million a year for 700 beds, or about $570,000 per bed. We are asked to believe that this amount of funding is insufficient to keep the place clean.

Although people may think that medical care has improved greatly since the 1950s, problems have been accumulating. The first alarm came with thalidomide, a tranquilizer prescribed to mothers-to-be for morning sickness. Thalidomide caused massive birth defects in babies who survived it, including drastic shortening of the arms, legs, or both. From 1957 to 1961, thalidomide was available in over 100 countries, in numerous medications with differing names. The United States was fortunate, in that approval of the drug was delayed and few children were born deformed. Despite this highly visible calamity, with thousands of deformed children around the world, it took time to discover the cause.[17] Thalidomide was a single high-profile drug that had exceptionally noticeable and debilitating side effects, and it was on the market for some years before its obvious problems became apparent. Currently, the extent of health degradation from drug side effects is not known.

Many hospital patients are given several drugs at the same time, a practice known as polypharmacy. This is risky, because as the number of drugs increases, the number of possible adverse interactions becomes large. One drug has zero interactions, two drugs have a single possible interaction with each other, three drugs have three interactions, four drugs have six interactions, and so on. Some patients are on ten or more drugs, and many patients risk fifty or more different interactions, the symptoms and effects of which are mostly unknown.

Medical science has no effective mechanism for investigating these numerous potential drug interactions. With each additional drug a patient takes, the possible side effects are multiplied. We are aware of cases where lowering the number of drugs has restored a person to health. When a patient is taking several drugs, it is difficult, if not impossible, to tell whether a symptom is caused by a disease or is a drug side effect.

Dr. Hickey had a relative who asked if he would review the possible side effects of her drugs. Alarmingly, she was taking thirteen prescription medications at the same time. There were seventy-eight direct interactions among the individual drugs and many more when groups of drugs were considered. The list of potential side effects of the individual drugs ran to many pages and it was not possible to determine the nature of the interactions. There was simply insufficient information in the scientific and medical literature to even make a reasonable guess at the side effects.

At this point, readers might consider that a gravely ill person entering hospital expects not to suffer an unnecessary "adverse event" that might further endanger their life. It is reasonable to assume that doctors will "first, do no harm." A one-in-fifty risk of death by treatment or error is unacceptable, whatever the circumstances. Transport provides a service and people accept that there is a small risk of injury or death when traveling, but few people would travel if the risk of injury or death were as high as two deaths or injuries in every 100 person-trips. Even Formula One racing drivers, extreme sports enthusiasts, or daredevil stunt drivers might not find that level of risk acceptable. Moreover, the service a hospital provides claims specifically to protect patients from illness and death, and return them to good health.

Dr. Lucian Leape[18] noted that autopsy has revealed potentially fatal misdiagnoses in 20–40 percent of cases.[19] Of people who died in a hospital and had an autopsy, roughly three in every ten might have been killed as a result of a faulty diagnosis. These figures are a low estimate of hospital errors, because a much higher proportion of people may have had adverse events that were not diagnosis-related or events that failed to be picked up at autopsy. We realize a diagnosis is the result of a decision-making process with much uncertainty. The patient, however, may still risk loss of a limb, or their life, when the diagnosis is wrong.

MEDICAL REGULATION

Governments have given the medical profession the right and duty to regulate itself, according to broad guidelines. Presumably, the reasoning is that only doctors have the necessary expertise. The aim is to protect the public against the ravages that might be caused by unethical, careless, or fraudulent doctors. There may, however, be another objective, which is seldom discussed—to protect the medical profession.

As we have described, medicine is the modern equivalent of a medieval European guild. These were powerful organizations and could kill a member who betrayed a guild secret. The guild was a trade association of craftsmen,[20] and early guilds were formed by groups of workers. They formed official cartels and were given authority to restrict trade to their members, an authority often based on charters or Letters Patent (*litterae patentes,* open letters) issued by the monarch. Further trade restrictions were achieved by limiting the supply of materials and tools. Guildhalls are still common in European towns as a continuing legacy.

An early example of the restrictive actions of a medical guild concerns the experiences of Thomas Sydenham (1624–1689), a lieutenant in Oliver Cromwell's army. After the English Civil War, Sydenham trained to become a doctor, eventually becoming known as the English Hippocrates. He completed his apprenticeship, passed his examinations, and was licensed by the London Medical Association.

In seventeenth-century England, the major disease was smallpox, which was thought to be caused by an excess of humors that the body was trying to eliminate. This explained both the pox, little volcano-like eruptions from the skin, and the fever. The conventional treatment had a long history, being established for at least 1,500 years: the aim was to increase the patient's fever to hasten the elimination of the noxious humors. Dr. Sydenham, like other doctors of the period, covered sufferers with blankets, closed windows, and administered whiskey. Since this was before the advent of central heating, it was particularly difficult to boost the fever in the cold winter.

Dr. Sydenham differed from his peers in that he counted the number of patients who died. According to theory, the death rate should have been higher in the winter than in the summer, as it was more difficult to increase the patients' temperature. To Sydenham's surprise, he found it was the other way around: the summer death rate was higher. This must have been puzzling and disturbing, but he believed what he saw rather than what the established theory proposed.

Dr. Sydenham decided to reverse his approach—in other words, to try and bring down the fever. He left patients uncovered, had them drink light English ale, and threw the windows open. The experiment worked: his summer death rate decreased to winter levels. We can imagine his state of mind: would we have the audacity to go counter to a theory that had been followed for over a thousand years? We all like to think we would have such intellectual courage, but, in reality, few are so reckless. After due deliberation, Dr. Sydenham made a grave mistake—he spoke out. The response was consistent with medicine throughout its history: the London Medical Association threatened to take away his license, while another doctor challenged him to a duel. Luckily, Dr. Sydenham had friends in high places. He wrote a letter to a member of the nobility, outlining his work and the problems he was facing. As he explained, "A medical discovery is like a sapling in the middle of the King's highway. If you do not fence it in, it will be trampled down by the galloping hoards." He was protected and later was even knighted.

Medical progress owes a great deal to such mavericks. Advances are made by people willing to go against the status quo and to challenge conventional clinical guidelines, if they are found to clash with experiment and direct observation.

Historically, the objective of a guild was to support its members, by holding secrets and protecting commercially valuable information. Nowadays, the medical establishment acts as a twenty-first century guild. While patents release information about drugs, practical knowledge and know-how is heavily restricted. When Dr. Hoffer studied medicine, it was fashionable to write prescriptions in Latin, denying patients knowledge of the substances that were being given. The establishment does more than try to impose restrictive practices—it also tries to prevent new ideas from being accepted. While it can no longer assassinate heretical members, it can destroy professional careers.

The eminent philosopher and Catholic priest, Ivan Illich, argues in his book *Limits to Medicine* that modern medicine does more damage than good.[21] Illich was one of the first to explain how modern medicine harms people by converting them into lifelong patients. To him, the institution of medicine was a conspiracy against people and their health. He was not being poetic or tangential—Illich meant what he wrote. He died after ten years of suffering cancer. He treated himself disregarding his doctor's advice to take a sedative, which would have prevented him from working. His views were largely ignored by medical authorities, who failed to provide an adequate response. Illich was not attacking medicine per se, but modern professions, which he considered to be much like medieval guilds. He could equally have attacked accountants or lawyers but chose medi-

Medical Nemesis

The defining moment in the realization that modern medicine could be harmful came in 1975 with the publication of Ivan Illich's book *Limits to Medicine: Medical Nemesis, The Expropriation of Health*.[22] "Expropriation" means the taking away or deprivation and a "nemesis" is a difficult-to-defeat enemy. Dr. Illich (1926–2002) argued that corporate medicine has turned against us and is literally depriving us of our health. He was a trained scientist and philosopher as well as a practicing Catholic priest. Rather appropriately, Illich describes doctors not as scientists but as medical clergy and their activities as disease producing (iatrogenic). He considered medicine to be a new religion that required faith and devotion from its followers, and that this medical monopoly was making us sick. His now classic book questions the outlook for anyone who contracts their health out to a doctor or hospital.

Ivan Illich considered modern medicine generally harmful. In his view, conventional medicine makes little contribution to life expectancy, has an insignificant effect on curing disease, and causes more illness than it alleviates.[23] By turning medicine into an industry, he suggests, physicians have removed responsibility for health from the individual. Illich has largely been ignored, though the twenty-first century provides several examples that support his contentions—in particular, the widespread reports of drug-resistant bacteria, such as MRSA and *Clostridium difficile*, a health care–associated intestinal infection. We agree with Illich that patients cannot rely on institutional medicine to minimize their health risks.

cine, presumably because it provided such a clear example of institutional misconduct.

CHANGING CLINICAL GUIDELINES

Throughout history, medical practitioners have claimed more than they could deliver. Even the most powerful have succumbed to medical ineptitude. The last words of Alexander the Great were "I am dying from the treatment of too many physicians." Alexander could conquer the world, but not his doctors. Modern patients are less influential, and the gradual process of turning healthy people into patients, as described by Ivan Illich, continues. One interesting feature of health guidelines is they gradually tighten; thus, healthy people are gradually redefined as sick. Classic examples are blood pressure and cholesterol levels.

Blood pressure is described as the maximum pressure (systolic or heart contraction) over the minimum pressure (diastolic or heart relaxation). Because the height of a mercury column was used in old blood pressure gauges, readings are written as millimeters of mercury (mm Hg). Normal ranges are 90–120 mm Hg (systolic) over 60–80 mm Hg (diastolic); an acceptable blood pressure might thus be stated as "120 over 80" and written as 120/80 mm Hg.

Blood pressure used to be considered high when the systolic pressure was consistently above 140 mm Hg. Recently, the values have been lowered and blood pressures above 115/75 mm Hg are considered a risk.[24] These pressures, formerly regarded as normal, convert healthy people into patients. Notably, despite the acknowledged connection between hypertension and diet, drugs are a primary intervention. Drugs to lower a person's blood pressure are prescribed for extended periods to treat this newly created chronic "disease," providing a steady income stream for the doctor and corporate medicine.

The real situation with blood pressure is rather complex. The published pressures are for resting individuals. If a person stands up, walks, runs, engages in conversation, or is stressed, the blood pressure rises. One form of stress is a doctor taking your blood pressure! Blood pressure readings are unreliable[25] and are often elevated during a medical examination, a phenomenon known as "white coat hypertension."[26] It is worth checking that your high blood pressure is not due to a white coat effect before going on a lifetime course of medication.

Similarly, cholesterol levels that were formerly considered normal are now thought by some to be dangerous. This example is slightly more difficult to assess. First, there is no evidence that cholesterol in the diet is harmful—this is a myth propagated quite recently by corporate medicine and the food industry. The body regulates blood cholesterol: if more cholesterol is consumed, the body simply makes less or breaks down more. The effect on blood levels is rather small. Furthermore, there is a scientific debate about blood cholesterol; specifically, the assumption that increased blood cholesterol increases the risk of atherosclerosis and heart attack is unsubstantiated.

As criticism of the cholesterol and heart disease hypothesis has increased, so the propagators of the cholesterol theory have adapted it. They claim it is not cholesterol in the diet or the blood that necessarily causes harm. Instead, they suggest there are both "good" and "bad" cholesterols in the blood. Supposedly, an imbalance between good and bad cholesterol is the source of the risk. As this idea is challenged, the circus moves on, and oxidized cholesterol becomes the latest culprit. We simply note that oxidized cholesterol is an indication of a shortage of antioxidants in the diet.[27]

Normal cholesterol levels are no longer accepted as healthy. We might ask, why does this matter? The reason is that many more people are defined as requiring expensive cholesterol-lowering drugs, such as statins. This increases the market, bringing normal people into the range for lifelong treatment. It has even been recommended that these drugs might be taken prophylactically, before there is any increase in cholesterol. Statin drugs have not been shown to save lives but do deplete the body of coenzyme Q_{10}, a molecule essential to every cell. Their use may cause chronic disease, but rigorous studies on long-term side effects will require decades. Such is the popularity of statins among a section of the medical establishment that some doctors have suggested, only half jokingly, that they might be added to the water supply. In the future, perhaps, our generation's cavalier use of statins might be regarded with the same horror that we reserve for bloodletting, leeches, and thalidomide.

EVIDENCE-BASED MEDICINE

Evidence-based medicine is the current fashion in medical research. The term *evidence-based* is a marketing dream, as obviously all medicine should be based on evidence—any other approach would be irrational. Archibald Cochrane, one of its pioneers, stated that medical interventions should be evaluated to make sure they are cost-effective and beneficial to the patient.[28] We agree with this notion, although not with the way it has been implemented.

Practicing medicine based on evidence is clearly a reasonable idea. However, this common sense interpretation is not what "evidence-based medicine" has come to mean. As currently practiced, this methodology refers largely to the use of certain limited statistics, population studies, and large-scale clinical trials. Medical scientists appear to believe that statistical medicine is, in some way, more powerful than direct scientific measurement, including physicians' own observations. Medical research depends hugely on statistics, despite the fact that many doctors are neither well trained nor interested in the decision sciences. David Wootton, author of *Bad Medicine,* went so far as to suggest that modern medicine is un-contentious as a result of its improving technology and the introduction of statistics.[29] Little could be further from the truth.

Modern medicine may have little influence of life span or well-being. The relatively recent increases in the human longevity and population size are partly a result of reductions in disease attributable to better nutrition and sanitation. Thomas McKeown studied influences on the world population from the eighteenth century to the 1970s.[30] He attributed improvements to social and economic changes rather than public health or medicine. Recently, researchers claimed that McKeown's conclusions had been discredited by subsequent research.[31] Needless to say, the research that purported to question McKeown was largely statistical in nature.[32] Critics claimed that the rise in population was largely due to an increase in birth rate rather than a fall in mortality.[33] The authors ask us to believe that McKeown's work can largely be dismissed as a historical footnote. However, this conclusion is irrational: the increased birthrate over this period was most likely driven by improved nutrition and sanitation, leading to increased survival of babies and children. Improved nutrition is a social change, which depends on economics. In dismissing McKeown's findings, these researchers wrongly attributed to medicine the credit due to agriculture, food, and social change.

Schoolboy Triumph

Considering the billions of dollars spent on medicine, hospitals, and related research, we might expect to be given reasonable advice on preventing illness. However, despite the hype, there is no incentive to provide real preventive medicine. We will illustrate the problem with the story of a schoolboy who instigated an official awareness campaign where medical organizations and corporate medicine had failed.

Fourteen-year-old Ryan McLaughlin lived in the Scottish city of Glasgow, which is not noted for its sunny climate.[34] His mother, Kirsten, had multiple sclerosis (MS) and Ryan had started showing symptoms of the disease. Then, the family visited sunny Australia, and his mother found that she was able to quit her wheelchair and get up and about, even practicing the martial art Tae Kwan Do. The family wondered what could be so helpful and decided it was sunlight. Intense sunlight generates large amounts of vitamin D in the skin. They looked into the literature and discovered evidence linking vitamin D to MS and other diseases, such as the flu and cancer. Kirsten started taking vitamin D supplements and her recovery continued.

Being a teenager was somewhat of an advantage, as Ryan gained backing from J. K. Rowling, author of the Harry Potter books. With the Multiple Sclerosis Society, they petitioned the Scottish government at Holyrood for free vitamin D to be provided to children and pregnant mothers. The government declined this suggestion but agreed to provide some official guidance on vitamin D. In Ryan's words, "I was shocked there had not been publicity around this before. We wanted there to be more awareness of the link and more research into how much of a problem it is in Scotland."

Why should it be left to the initiative of a schoolboy to acknowledge the relationship between MS and vitamin D? This is one disease and one vitamin, but there are numerous other illnesses that vitamin D will prevent. And vitamin D is only a single nutrient; inadequate intake of nutrients is a feature of diseases from arthritis to zoster (shingles).

Surprisingly, doctors are likely to tell you vitamins can cause more harm than good. If they do, remember that doctor may have less knowledge in this area than a fourteen-year-old schoolboy.

CONFLICTS OF INTEREST

Conflict of interest is inherent in the practice of medicine. Doctors are paid for treating patients; if there were no sick people, there would be no medical profession. A psychiatrist who treats patients with psychotherapy each week is financially rewarded for each visit. If another doctor cures the patient after just one visit, the second doctor's financial reward will be correspondingly small. Thus, effective medicine can hurt a doctor's pocket. The ineffective doctor will be financially secure, while the good doctor will struggle to survive. Similarly, if they treated patients successfully, hospitals could go broke. An epidemic of health could have severe economic consequences for some.

Often there is no financial incentive to cure or to prevent chronic conditions. Preventive medicine is even less rewarding than providing a cure. Public health doctors, who carry out research into disease prevention, are mostly salaried—they get paid whether they succeed or not. Moreover, it can require powerful social action to introduce preventive health measures. For example, 100 years ago, in the southeast United States, there were prolonged outbreaks of pellagra, a disease characterized by four D's—dermatitis, diarrhea, dementia, and death. Shortage of niacin (vitamin B_3) made people sick and psychotic, but this was not known at the time; the disease was attributed to other causes, such as spoiled corn or infection.

In some years, the disease struck as many as 300,000 people and helped fill mental hospitals. In 1914, Dr. Joseph Goldberger was invited to head the Public Health Service's pellagra investigations. He noticed that pellagra occurred among the inmates of mental institutions but did not affect the nurses and attendants. He therefore hypothesized that pellagra was a dietary disease since, if it were an infection, the care staff would be expected to catch it.

To test his idea, Drs. Goldberger and George Wheeler fed volunteers a monotonous diet of white bread and similar refined food to see if this would produce pellagra.[35] The pellagra squad, who consumed the restricted diet, were twelve volunteers from the Mississippi State Penitentiary; they agreed on the basis that they would receive a pardon; 108 control convicts were given an enhanced diet, including meat and dairy foods. After six months, six of the pellagra squad developed pellagra, while none of the controls developed the disease.

To counter the notion that pellagra was caused by an infectious agent, Dr. Goldberger went even further. In what they called "filth parties," he, his wife, and several others inoculated themselves with the blood, feces, urine, and other secretions of the sick. They applied these samples up the nose and in the mouth, as well as by injection. None of these volunteers became ill. Later, Goldberger produced the equivalent disease to human pellagra (known as black tongue) in dogs by restricting their diet.

Despite Dr. Goldberger's daring experiments, opposition to his dietary theory of pellagra continued. Physicians clung to their view that infection was the cause, and politicians were outraged by the suggestion that their area was poor and in need of social reform. Dr. Goldberger's wife, Mary, a grandniece of Confederate President Jefferson Davis, was particularly unhappy at the opposition her husband faced after he discovered that pellagra was a deficiency disease and showed how to prevent and cure it.

Sadly, Dr. Goldberger died in 1929 before his findings were finally implemented. In the decade following his death, Dr. Tom Spies and others showed that niacin (vitamin B_3) cured pellagra in humans. During World War Two, the U.S. government authorized the addition of vitamin B_3 to flour and the pandemic vanished, one of the most successful public health preventive measures.

The strange reluctance of medicine to embrace nutrition continues to this day. Health authorities preach contradictory viewpoints. People are advised to eat five helpings of fruit and vegetables a day to prevent disease and stay healthy. Yet, even though nutritional deficiency is apparently accepted as a cause of disease, modern medicine claims that the sick will achieve little benefit from nutritional supplementation. Doctors accept a strange form of double think, whereby nutrition is both a primary determinant of health and of little benefit to their patients.

Physicians know about past advances from improved nutrition, such as prevention of pellagra, rickets, and scurvy. They are less aware that these developments arose in the face of vehement opposition from medical authorities. Many still believe, as doctors have through the ages, that medicine has changed and has become more scientific. However, although corporate medicine has introduced new technologies, the primary economic paradigm remains: patients are the doctors' raw material, and disease prevention or cure reduces the supply of patients on whom to practice.

Dishonesty

People, doctors included, are not always honest. When publishing a research paper in a medical journal, doctors are often asked to declare any financial interests. The journal's aim is to reduce the frequency of publishing what looks like a valid research paper but is in reality little more than advertising copy for a medical product. However, the value of the declaration depends on the doctor giving an honest and accurate response, which is often not the case. A second doctor reading the article would like to know if the authors have any financial interests in the treatment. The readers' view of the results might be quite different if the authors stand to make large amounts of money from the success of the drug or equipment.

John Fauber, a reporter at the *Milwaukee Journal Sentinel,* investigated the accuracy of self-declared interests.[36] Fauber found that nine doctors at the University of Wisconsin Medical School incorrectly declared they had no conflict of interest when publishing papers. They told the journal that they had no conflicts of interest or relationship with companies that had a financial interest in their work.

Consider one example. In 2008, Dr. M, a cancer specialist, wrote an article for the *International Journal of Radiation Oncology-Biology-Physics,* which offers authoritative articles linking new research and technologies to clinical applications. The paper was about therapeutic results obtained using radiation equipment manufactured by a local company. However, Dr. M was a paid consultant to the company that developed the equipment described in the study; the other authors declared that they had related interests, but Dr. M did not. Dr. M could have made a mistake. Fauber found that before Dr. M submitted his paper, he told the university that he was working as a consultant to the technology firm. As a result, he was lowering his working involvement with the university. He admitted that he would receive more than $20,000 in addition to $10,000 worth of stock options. The reporter discovered that, in 2008, Dr. M received $75,000 from the company for twenty days' consultancy. The value of his stock options also increased.

The presence and influence of corporate medicine pushes treatment rather than prevention. Doctors typically have sufficient patients with an adequate number of diseases to keep them busy. There would appear to be no reason for preventive medicine to be unpopular. However, to corporate medicine, patients and diseases provide profits. A medical company is expected to grow and increase profits to a maximum for its shareholders. In so doing, the company is not being unethical—it is fulfilling its legal reason for existence.

There are times in medicine when calculated risks are unavoidable. However, this should always be the patient's decision. For example, a new operation has to be tried on that first patient. As in any operation, the surgeon should explain the procedure and risks involved. Often, however, the risks are not known—the surgeon cannot know the risks of an operation that has never been performed. In such cases, a surgeon might have many influences beyond the health of the patient. The new operation may help the patient, but on the other hand, it could kill him or her; the surgeon obviously hopes the patient will benefit. In addition, other people could be helped by the procedure. Furthermore, success may advance the surgeon's career, allowing him or her to present at a prestigious conference or get a promotion. The surgeon might hold a patent on a piece of novel technology required for the operation. In other words, the surgeon could be subject to conflicts of interest. There are good reasons why the patient should decide whether or not to undergo the surgery, after being given access to all the relevant information. All too often, patients are involved in trials whose main purpose is to benefit medicine rather than the individual.

WISHFUL THINKING

Throughout history, medicine has been dominated by wishful thinking and irrationality. People are subject to irrational confirmation bias and doctors are no exception. They prefer information that supports their prejudices, so doctors look for data and research results that confirm their pre-existing ideas, and they avoid information that contradicts their prejudice. When a report disagrees with the current opinions, they are likely to find an argument why the experiment was invalid, denigrate the experiment, or malign the scientist. This defensive posture was applied to pioneers of orthomolecular medicine. Even Linus Pauling was called a quack when he suggested that the data on vitamin C and prevention of disease needed serious consideration. If that can happen to one of the most successful scientists in history, do not expect prejudiced doctors to treat you as an equal.

When a patient gets better, the doctor takes the credit—clearly, the treatment worked. An old joke is that the operation was successful, but the patient died. It took many years of failed operations before open heart surgery was practicable. The pioneering heart surgeons gained prestige, promotion, and fame for their successes;[37] failures were ignored once people began to survive the procedure. But the early open heart patients often died or were disabled. In effect, these patients sacrificed their lives for the eventual benefit of others. However, while they might have suggested this was an altruistic outcome, wishful thinking may have led to their sacrifice. Like doctors, patients suffer from a positive outcome bias: they are not rational, but focus on the chance that things will go their way.

Patients believe a positive outcome is more likely than a negative one, irrespective of the probabilities. A common example is that a person often imagines winning the lottery, but the risk of dying in an automobile accident is ignored. Of course, rationally, death by motor vehicle is far more likely than becoming an overnight lottery millionaire. One idea provides hope and good feeling, while the other fear and despair.

Back in 1929, Dr. F. H. Garrison thought modern scientific medicine was fine—medicine had changed since the barbaric old days.[38] A similar assertion is made by Dr. Druin Burch's recent book on evidence-based medicine, *Taking the Medicine*.[39] On the back cover is the following statement: "Doctors have unwittingly killed rather than healed. This book shows how that happened, and how we can stop it in the future." In his final chapter, Dr. Burch quotes Lewis Thomas, who qualified in medicine in 1937, as finding that, despite sulfonamides, contemporary hospitals offered little more to the sick than hotel accommodation. "Whether you survived or not depended on the natural history of the disease itself," wrote Lewis. "Medicine made little or no difference."

Dr. Burch goes on to claim that "randomized controlled trials have swept away much suffering and error from hospitals and homes, ushering in comfort and healing instead." A few lines before this, he mentions without irony that "there is a bitter joke in medicine: the violence with which someone makes an argument is inversely proportional to the amount of evidence they have backing it up. The more people are left without reliable experiments, the more they seem to fall back on strongly held opinions, as though confidence was a starch that could stiffen ideas into facts simply by being applied with enough fervor." Dr. Burch himself is clearly fervent in his appreciation of randomized, controlled trials, though the evidence is that suffering and error still blight our hospitals.

CHAPTER 3

Poor Hospital Management

*"Those who think they have no time for healthy eating
will sooner or later have to find time for illness."*
—EDWARD STANLEY (1826–1893)

We are told that modern medicine is scientific and that advances in technology provide the patient with greater potential for a return to health. In part, this is true: properly employed, modern medical technology has many advantages, particularly for diagnosis and surgery. However, the technology is poorly utilized and hospitals cause harm as a result of inadequate practice and management.

A sick person goes to the doctor for help, receives treatment, and, typically, returns to health. However, most illnesses resolve naturally within a limited time and people return to relative well-being, whether they are treated or not. In some cases, hospitals are essential: emergency medicine can heal people when they have suffered major trauma. A diabetic can receive insulin, which will overcome the acute risk of coma and death. Surgeons can remove an infected appendix and, potentially, save a life. There are numerous benefits of modern medicine. These examples do not, however, answer the question of whether hospitals provide an overall benefit.

As we have explained, each year hospitals are known to kill or harm many thousands of patients; many more people suffer serious or fatal drug side effects. We need to balance the benefits provided by modern medicine against these unnecessary deaths, and it is not clear that modern medicine helps more people than it harms. We need to know, for example, whether doctors prevent more deaths with antibiotics each year than are killed by drug-resistant bacteria and other hospital-acquired infections.

49

Hospitals should exist for the benefit of patients. Despite this, management, technology, and treatment methods seem to take precedence. This phenomenon is not new—it began long ago and increases with the advancement of technology. When the stethoscope was introduced, it separated the doctor from the patient. Previously, doctors listened with their ears pressed against the chest or back of the patient. French doctor René Laennec (1781–1826) invented the stethoscope. He noticed some children playing with a stick that transmitted the sound of a scratching pin. His first instrument was a rolled up piece of paper, but it worked. However, some could see this was the beginning of technological separation of physician from patient. Dr. Robert Volz (1806-1882), a German physician, remarked that "the sick have become a thing."[1] The introduction of anesthesia into surgery greatly reduced the suffering that patients previously endured. However, it meant that the unconscious patients were completely at the mercy of the surgeon. In a sense, a surgical patient is a thing, an object to be acted upon. An anesthetized patient does not complain.

As medical technology has advanced, so has the professional management of hospitals. Patients may now be referred to as "clients" or even as "cost centers." Productivity and cost effectiveness are now considered essential. Even if such labels are applied to the stream of patients entering and leaving the hospital, their individual needs should still take precedence over management tools.

Hospitals have changed dramatically in the last few decades. By the 1970s, U.S. hospitals were ceasing to be places where private doctors cared for their private patients. The hospital as an organization began to assume comprehensive responsibility for the total health care of patients.[2] This increase in scope came without a corresponding enhancement of management.

Problems associated with poor management and inadequate treatment occur in many countries, and they extend from developing countries to the most advanced intensive care units. Africa is beset with an epidemic of AIDS, which is blamed on unsafe sexual practices. However, we are not often told that one in five of the new cases of HIV infection occur as a result of inappropriate medical intervention.[3] Reusing hypodermic needles may appear to be cost saving but risks spreading infection. Over a quarter of adults diagnosed with HIV in South Africa had not had recent sexual encounters.[4] Furthermore, over one in six HIV-positive children had

HIV-negative mothers.[5] Local politicians and health managers underesti-
mate hospital-induced HIV infection, as it exonerates them from responsibility.[6] Public health managers do not inform Africans about the risk of
unsafe health care.[7] No African government has examined medically
caused HIV infection by tracing those who went to suspected clinics. In
short, medical practice is inadvertently promoting HIV infection in Africa.
The standard response to the shortcomings of medicine in developing
countries is to suggest additional funding to provide proper medical care.

Even the most technically advanced and well-funded clinics can be as
dangerous as medical care in the Third World. Hospital managers in
advanced countries are simply better at hiding the issues. Here, for comparison, are two problems in intensive care units worldwide:

- The risk of a person in intensive care being infected with by a life-threatening bug is about 50/50. Of 13,796 patients in intensive care, half
  (7,087) were infected.[8]

- The longer a person was in intensive care, the more likely they were to
  be infected. This was especially true for antibiotic-resistant superbugs.
  Most patients (9,084) were on antibiotics.

Importantly, the death rate for infected patients (25 percent) was more
than double that of non-infected patients (11 percent).

Comparison of figures for intensive care unit infections in North America and Africa is instructive. North American infection rates were slightly
below the international average, at 48 percent.[9] However, the lowest rate
of infection was in Africa, at 46 percent. Moreover, the overall infection
rates appear to have increased from 45 percent in 1995 to 51 percent
today. Poor management is a characteristic of modern medical practice,
and this involves a number of fundamental structural problems.

LACK OF BASIC EXPERTISE AND EQUIPMENT

Poor management of hospitals is a primary cause of death and suffering.
The British Government conducted a review of the care of patients who
died within four days of entering hospital.[10] It would appear that people
working in hospitals often lacked basic expertise. They noted that some
health-care professionals did not have the skills required to care for
patients nearing the end of their lives. They lacked ability to identify

patients who were near death, gave inadequate care to the dying, and lacked basic communication skills.

In a quarter of the patients who died (407/1,635), there was a delay in being seen by a consultant. One in seven (267/1,983) clinical teams had inadequate communication with each other and with other medical groups. Doctors with different levels of authority did not talk to each other. Decision making was poor and there was a lack of support from senior doctors, especially during the night shifts. Over 4 percent of patients who were anesthetized were put under by an unsuitable doctor.

For patients entering the hospital with a life-threatening condition, access to medical imaging is a primary requirement. However, the government report noted that only about half the hospitals (150/297) had on-site non-cardiac angiography (medical imaging of blood vessels). Moreover, only about one hospital in four had 24-hour angiography available.

Similarly, there was inadequate access to computerized tomography (CT) and magnetic resonance imaging (MRI) scans in many hospitals. Even in those hospitals with advanced imaging facilities, they may not be available outside of office hours. Some time ago, Dr. Hickey worked in a medical school, investigating the physics of one of the early MRI scanners. At that time, there were few operational MRI scanners and the equipment was used almost exclusively for research. However, the hospital next door was fundraising for a new scanner. They could have used the one in the medical school for urgent patients, when it was not being used for research. When Dr. Hickey suggested the idea, it was refused on the grounds that nursing cover was not available. However, the suggestion was not put to the hospital management, who might have been able to provide nurses in the interim, until they had raised the millions of dollars necessary for their own MRI unit.

Smaller local hospitals have particular difficulties as they lack expertise and management. Providing a high standard of care for sick children requires well managed clinical teams. A particular concern is limitation of treatment. Doctors may engage in so-called heroic methods to keep a dying person alive. It is difficult to see how such a term can be applied. It is the patient who is in danger, not the doctors. With those patients not expected to survive, 16.9 percent (219/1,293) had no evidence of any discussion of limiting the care with the relatives or with the patient. Where a "do not resuscitate" (DNR) order was implemented, 21.8 percent were signed by trainee doctors.

NO CONTINUITY OF CARE

Many hospitals in the United Kingdom used to have health professionals with specific responsibility for a patient's care, and the patient felt they had a relationship with their doctors and nurses. In those days, doctors had a clear accountability for the health of patients. However, recent changes in hospital management have changed the structure of clinical teams. The patient may see a doctor infrequently, and they may not see the same doctor twice. The National Confidential Enquiry into Patient Outcome and Death noted, "Individual clinicians become transient acquaintances during a patient's illness rather than having responsibility for continuity of care."[11] This lack of both the personal touch and continuity of treatment may be expected to occur with the changes in the U.S. health-care system.

Poor management and accountability are a major cause of dissatisfaction, appropriate treatment, and patient death. The reported results are terrible. According to Katherine Murphy, from the Patients Association, they result in "life-threatening complications left untreated, poor note keeping, seriously ill patients deteriorating without prompt action, lack of facilities for emergency surgery, avoidable complications contributing to patient death."[12]

In four out of ten severely ill patients, the standard of care is appalling. This has consequences beyond the direct effects on the patient. Relatives, those nearest to the dying patients, are not only bereaved but can have dreadful memories of what happened. Palliative care is the minimum for a dying patient: it is not intended to cure but to minimize symptoms and make the patient comfortable.[13] However, the minimum requirements for palliative care, to relieve pain and other distressing symptoms, are not being achieved in hospitals.

The problems are becoming widespread and apparent. Vincent Nichols, the Archbishop of Westminster, recently described hospital care of some patients as "lacking in humanity."[14] Those in need of care and attention were treated as "a bundle of genes and actions," according to the Archbishop. "Even the most restricted of lives is lived in transcendence by virtue of being human. If we fail to see this and honor it, then we not only fail to respect a person: we do that person violence." The cleric also identifies the problem as being a result of the organization and not individual doctors and nurses: "It is not simply a matter of the attitudes of individuals, though of course that is part of the story. It is also about the prevailing culture in an institution, the pressures of control and delivery which can impair and diminish the ability of staff to care properly." What was missing, said the Archbishop, was "a sense of humility, a profound respect for others, and a refusal to see them as no more than a medical or behavioral problem to be tackled and resolved."

SECRECY THAT HIDES INEPTITUDE

The secrecy surrounding bad management in medicine is pathogenic. The role of medical confidentiality is to protect patients, but it can also be used to cover up incompetence by hospital staff.[15] A patient's details and discussion of their health with their physician is protected by law. Historically, this confidentiality goes back at least as far as Hippocrates. However, there are limits that vary with the local laws:

- In the U.S., gunshot wounds are customarily reported to the police.

- People unfit to drive a motor vehicle may be similarly reported.

- The spouse may be informed of a partner's sexually transmitted disease.[16]

Despite these limitations, confidentiality is necessary for trust in the doctor-patient relationship.[17] Nurses and paramedics have a similar duty of secrecy. Health professionals frequently need to communicate a patient's confidential details to other care workers in order to provide adequate treatment. Those patients with particular concerns may need to request constraints on this sharing of data as confidential information leaks occasionally to the detriment of the patient.[18]

Wherever there is confidentiality, professionals can keep secrets to protect themselves. Such secrecy hides wrongdoing and ineptitude. This extends to professionals who use confidentiality to shield colleagues from the consequences of their actions. Moreover, medical organizations can use secrecy to cover negligence and overcharging.

Human Error

Most hospital accidents are the result of human error. Doctors, nurses, and other health professionals are as prone to making mistakes as the rest of us. Unfortunately, the result of their errors can be catastrophic: often a patient suffers a serious adverse event, or even dies. People sometimes compare hospitals with the airline travel industry. In both, there is a risk to life, but there the similarity ends. When an airplane crashes, hundreds of people may be killed and the world media reports the accident in detail. By contrast, medicine kills at least the equivalent of a major air crash each day, but the deaths are rarely reported. Moreover, through consistent checks and monitoring, air travel has become remarkably safe. Conversely, medicine remains responsible for hundreds of thousands of deaths each year.

The defense of modern medicine is typically based on the assumption that it does more good than harm. If you are unfortunate enough to be involved in an airplane crash or, more likely, a car accident, the hospital is there to pick up the pieces. Without a hospital, far more people would die or be permanently disabled from such events. But the majority of people treated in hospital do not fall into this category and are not in immediate risk of dying—except from the treatment and care provided.

Power Relationships

The aircraft and travel industries have addressed and reduced the errors that endanger passenger lives. Engineering problems were relatively straightforward: imposition of quality control into manufacture and maintenance means that aircraft seldom fall from the sky as a result of mechanical failure. Nowadays, as with unnecessary hospital deaths, air crashes are largely the result of human error. Typically, a crash follows from a sequence of errors, each of which does not inevitably threaten the aircraft, but a combination of five or more errors may be disastrous.

Between 1970 and 1999, Korean Air crashed 16 aircraft, with the loss of 700 lives. Malcolm Gladwell, in his book *Outliers*, describes how Korean Air turned this unacceptably high accident rate around.[19] Interestingly, they did this by addressing the hierarchical social structure of the cabin crew. To avoid a crash, co-pilots and engineers are required to check the captain's decisions and actions. A pilot may be tired or may simply miss a cockpit warning sign. Co-pilots are also responsible for communicating with ground controllers and pilots. Communication in the aircraft cabin needs to be clear and direct. A statement like "The aircraft is too low, pull up" is a clear instruction to the pilot. It tells the captain to increase altitude and provides a reason. However, if the co-pilot says, "Are we a little low?" this is more of a question, which does not demand any immediate action. If the plane is in danger, the co-pilot needs to declare the problem and action clearly.

In cultures such as that of Korea, which have a high degree of respect for authority, a suggestion is more acceptable than a straightforward instruction. Within Korean Air, the social structure in the cockpit was hierarchical. Co-pilots and flight engineers were loathe to make demands of the superior captain or to highlight even the most obvious errors. The solution was to change the culture in the cockpit, so that co-pilots and engineers were able to correct pilot error and communicate effectively with ground control. Staff received training courses to reduce their sense of deference, as a result of which the accident rate was greatly reduced.

The safety record of the air travel industry has a direct message for medicine.[20] Dr. Geert Hofstede, an influential Dutch psychologist, introduced the idea of a power distance. This measures how much members of institutions and organizations expect and accept the unequal distribution of power.[21] Culture can influence the behavior of professionals and generate a risk of error.[22] In low power distance organizations, people consider themselves more or less equal in status, regardless of their formal positions. In high power distance organizations, members have great respect for authority and for the power it provides. Korean Air staff originally had a high power distance, which was lowered through training, thus increasing safety.

In general, professions have relatively level hierarchies. A flat hierarchy is essential if an educated professional is to have the individual authority necessary to do their work.[23] Hospitals, however, are an extreme case—power relationships dominate the professional function. In other words, hospitals have a high power distance. In the past, this was so obvious that it formed the basis of doctor jokes and comedy. For example, "What is the difference between God and a consultant surgeon?" Answer, "God doesn't think he's a surgeon!"

There is a strict hierarchy between members of the medical professions. This has nothing to do with the teaching element. Hospital staff may explain that their authority is essential to the therapeutic process: patients need to have faith in their doctor. Thus, the doctor needs to be authoritative to put the patient's mind at rest. Patients like to feel that the surgeon about to operate on them is a senior professional with a high level of competence. Alternatively, they may claim that the placebo effect may be more effective if the patient respects the position of the doctor. This is, of course, special pleading and nonsense. Doctors and surgeons are expected to be competent because of their training and knowledge. Wearing a white coat and being pompous does not help to heal patients.

The order of status in the medical profession is attending surgeon, fellow, chief resident, and resident. For nurses, it is nurse manager, resource nurse, charge nurse, and staff nurse.[24] However, this description ignores the patients. Patients and their relatives are the lowest level in this power structure. Often, the "clients" are called by their first name. This may be the case even if the patient is a doctor, a professor, or a retired surgeon. We have seen junior nurses calling an internationally famous professor, who had the misfortune to become an inpatient, by her first name.

The hierarchy is so pervasive that it extends to the diseases a doctor treats.[25] Among specialties, neurosurgery and thoracic surgery have the highest rank, while geriatrics has a low rank. A doctor will be proud of the status of treating heart attacks, leukemia, and brain tumors, but may be less forthcoming about a specialization in fibromyalgia or anxiety neurosis.

The hierarchy in medicine is destructive to the health of patients. A young doctor who openly corrects a consultant or attending physician is unlikely to prosper in his or her career. Constructive criticism by a student doctor is considered whistle-blowing.[26] Nurses are trained to be subservient to doctors, so there is little chance for effective feedback to prevent accidents. A doctor who insists on professional dominance over patients and other staff is a threat to their health.[27] One educated patient we know was prepared for a hip operation, but they marked the wrong leg. He did not ask why they were marking his left leg, when the bad hip was in the right leg—presumably, he had been conditioned to assume the staff knew what they were doing. Fortunately, they noticed the mistake shortly before the operation, avoiding a catastrophe. These kinds of errors are not always caught in time.

One of the steps Korean Air took was to insist that cockpit staff use first names for all their colleagues. This was to help level the distribution of power. In non-clinical university departments, it is common for all to use their first names. The most renowned professor might be called "Jane" by John, a first-year student. The distinction between staff and students is clear, but not explicitly enforced, and there is no apparent loss of respect in this low power distance approach. The professor's respect is based on merit. Clinical units, however, often insist on titles.

We suggest that patients insist on being called by their formal title, say, "Mr. Smith." If the hospital staff decide to use your first name, then demand to use theirs. Being a physician does not allow him or her to be disrespectful to patients. Make sure you do not allow medical staff to assume authority over you. This is not arrogance, it is a matter of safety— when doctors and nurses assume an unwarranted authority, patients suffer.

Obedience to Authority

Although each of us must ultimately make our decisions alone, it is our nature to pay attention to input from others, especially those in authority. In Stanley Milgram's famous experiment in the 1970s, white-coated authority figures were able to get subjects to deliver apparently painful and possibly deadly shocks to other human beings, simply because they were told to.[28] A surprising number of reasonably intelligent people automatically defer to authority figures, and this is the case even when the authority figure is clearly wrong or immoral.

People can find it difficult to tell the difference between stupid obedience to authority and thinking for themselves. We all tend to believe we would question authority and not shock strangers or commit other unspeakable acts. The facts are generally less flattering. Charles Hofling, a psychiatrist, did a study on the obedience of nurses, with disturbing results.[29] Twenty-two hospital nurses were telephoned by people claiming to be doctors and were asked to give a drug overdose to a patient. The "doctor" said he was running late and would be along later to complete the paperwork. They were asked to give a dose of 20 mg of Astrofen, a phony drug that had been placed on the ward. The drug was clearly labeled with a safe maximum dose of only 10 mg. Remarkably, twenty-one nurses were willing to administer the drug overdose. They did not know the caller, other than that he claimed to be a doctor, and his request broke the rules of prescribing: the drug was not on the list of drugs to be administered. Importantly, Hofling asked twenty-two control nurses what they would do in this situation, and all but one said they would refuse the order. In other words, most people do not do what they think they would do. In medicine, unwarranted obedience to authority is pernicious and can cost lives.

OUT OF CONTROL

Hospitals work with dangerous medical interventions, which require controls to prevent error. Even in diagnostic areas, lack of control systems can cause harm. X-rays, as most people are aware, have the side effect of increasing cancer risk. X-ray CT body scans expose the body to large amounts of radiation and should be avoided, unless essential. A current fashion is to use whole-body scans to screen apparently healthy people to prevent disease. However, even the U.S. Food and Drug Administration (FDA) can find no justification or benefit for subjecting healthy people to the large dose of x-rays in a typical body scan.[30] Anyone who undergoes such screening increases their risk of cancer and of being treated unnecessarily for a benign condition. In getting normal controls for brain scanning on an early MRI system, two out of twenty-four normal subjects were found by Dr. Hickey's group to have abnormal brains. The abnormalities were causing no apparent symptoms and the decision was made not to inform the volunteers. However, if a harmless lump or abnormality is found in screening, you may be advised to have exploratory surgery or removal of the tissue. Such health screening is irrational, as it does not balance the possible benefits against the known risks.[31]

Even when equipment is working properly, mismanagement can cause unnecessary danger to patients. As well as the inherent risk of a standard head or body scan, failure to set up a scanner correctly can expose patients to risk. In February 2008, technicians at Cedars-Sinai Medical Center in Los Angeles did not set up the equipment properly for a new brain scan protocol.[32] The scanner was going to be used to image blood flow in the brain to help assess stroke patients. Unfortunately, an administrative error with the instructions led to the default settings being used and about eight times the intended radiation was delivered to the patients. The problem was noticed in August of the following year, when a stroke patient complained that he was losing his hair as a result of the scan. As a result, and to avoid the problem of widespread error in CT scanning control, the FDA issued a warning to hospitals.[33] The FDA suggested that radiological staff should note the dose indicator on the control panel!

Lack of a simple checklist is causing thousands of people to suffer botched operations. Hospitals could prevent four in ten surgical deaths if staff followed basic safety rules. Similarly, three in ten surgical complications would be avoided.[34] The World Health Organization (WHO) has developed such a checklist. The WHO questions are quite basic and relate to having the correct patient, staff, and equipment:

Before anesthesia:
- Has the patient confirmed his/her identity, site, procedure, and consent?
- Is the site marked?
- Is the anesthesia machine and medication check complete?
- Is the pulse oximeter on the patient and functioning?
- Does the patient have a known allergy?
- Is there a difficult airway or aspiration risk?
- Is there risk of greater than 500 ml (7 ml/kg in children) blood loss?

Before cutting the patient:
- Confirm all team members have introduced themselves by name and role.
- Confirm the patient's name, procedure, and where the incision will be made.
- Has antibiotic prophylaxis been given within the last sixty minutes?

   For surgeon:
   - What are the critical or non-routine steps?
   - How long will the case take?
   - What is the anticipated blood loss?

   For anesthetist:
   - Are there any patient-specific concerns?

At end of operation:

   For nursing team:
   - Has sterility (including indicator results) been confirmed?
   - Are there equipment issues or any concerns?
   - Is essential imaging displayed?

   Nurse verbally confirms:
   - The name of the procedure
   - Completion of instrument, sponge, and needle counts
   - Specimen labeling (read specimen labels aloud, including patient name)
   - Whether there are any equipment problems to be addressed

To surgeon, anesthetist, and nurse:
o What are the key concerns for recovery and management of this patient?

These simple rules would save numerous lives. The sorts of errors that are to be avoided include operating on the wrong patient. Richard Reznick, Head of Surgery at the University of Toronto, investigated the checklist in order to set an international standard. Dr. Reznick collected information on complications and deaths in 7,688 surgical patients who underwent surgery in centers throughout the world (Amman, Auckland, Ifakara, London, Manila, New Delhi, Seattle, and Toronto). The hospitals adopted the WHO checklist to determine if it would lower the number of complications and deaths. Complications occurred in 11 percent (411/3,733) of patients who had surgery before the checklists were used; 56 of the patients died. With the checklist, complications occurred in only 7 percent (277/3,955) of patients; only 32 patients died. This is a *substantial* improvement. Similar management controls on infection would bring the death rate down further.

These checklists highlight a fundamental problem with corporate medicine: basic rules of management control are absent. Most organizations in order to be successful need to implement feedback mechanisms to prevent errors, mistakes, and accidents. What few attempts there have been to introduce proper controls into medicine have been rudimentary and ineffective. If an elementary checklist can save lives, proper management controls might revolutionize hospitals into the centers of excellence they claim to be.

Hospitals need to take greater care with patient safety. The sort of management controls that are currently proposed are a minimum that would be anticipated in any industry. Other industries such as air and rail travel are expected to take measures for the safety of the public for whom they have a direct responsibility. Hospitals are a special case, where people are at their most vulnerable, and they have a particular responsibility for the health and well-being of the sick. As Phil Bronstein, a journalist who led an investigation by Hearst media, put it, "The annual medical error death toll is higher than that for fatal car crashes."[35] It is not acceptable for the number of unnecessary deaths to have increased over the last ten years.

IMPROVING MANAGEMENT TO PREVENT ERROR

Some errors will happen in any human activity. However, medical errors have serious consequences and, importantly, most are relatively easy to prevent. A crucial improvement in hospital management would be to identify problem areas and avoid consequent errors. In particular, the central role in preventing errors is to place the control with the doctor-patient or nurse-patient interaction. The educated people providing care could help prevent these errors, given the opportunity. Central management and control leads to waste, inefficiency, and, in the case of medicine, dead patients.

Management science has improved over recent decades and has achieved a startling reduction in manufacturing errors. To put the hospital problem into perspective, a Boeing 747 Jumbo Jet has approximately 6 million parts, about half of which are fasteners, 171 miles of wiring, and a typical flight has 50,000 service items.[36] Just as doctors are responsible for the safety of their patients, aircraft companies have to protect passengers. Every flight involves a risk to hundreds of passengers. However, compared to spending a day being treated in a hospital, the risk associated with flying is minute.

The failure of hospitals to protect patients stands out in our safety-conscious world. In manufacturing, Boeing and other aircraft companies follow strict practices of quality control, such as those pioneered by the American statistician William Edward Deming.[37] It was Dr. Deming whose ideas turned "made in Japan" from an indication of shoddy goods to a validation of quality. Japanese business embraced his ideas, while the rest of the world largely ignored them. Dr. Deming found that by implementing principles of management, organizations can simultaneously increase quality *and* reduce costs. In manufacturing, a company could reduce waste and rework, while enhancing customer loyalty. Similarly, hospitals and other organizations could avoid staff attrition and patient litigation as side effects of appropriate quality control. The aim is to think of the hospital and treatment as a (cybernetic) system, not as ad hoc individual parts. Continuous monitoring and improvement are key elements of the process.

Currently, if an error occurs, there is a good chance the hospital will not tell the patient. This is regrettable, as the key to real quality is negative feedback. In this context, negative feedback does not just mean complaints—it means recognizing the error and taking action to stop it from happening again. Unfortunately, in recent times, doctors and hospitals have developed a not-unfounded fear of litigation. Lawyers advise them to deny and defend: do not admit the error and refer to a lawyer. This is presumably an excellent source of income for the legal profession, but it prevents progress, as the feedback loop is blocked.

Das Gupta took a different approach.[38] He had inadvertently taken a piece of tissue from the patient's ninth rib rather than the eighth. In many years of practice, he had never made this mistake before. Dr. Gupta told the patient, "After all these years, I cannot give you any excuse whatsoever. . . . It is just one of those things that occurred. I have to some extent harmed you." The case was settled amicably.

Two U.S. universities and the U.K. National Health Service[39] have taken up the challenge of admitting errors and apologizing. Since their initiative, the University of Michigan Health System's monthly claims and lawsuits have declined; for example, from 262 in August 2001 to 83 in August 2007. This reduction could have been a direct result of the disclosure or because of improvements to safety. In the words of the risk officer, Richard C. Boothman, "Improving patient safety and patient communication is more likely to cure the malpractice crisis than defensiveness and denial." The hospital's claims and legal costs dropped to two-thirds of previous levels. Similarly, the number of malpractice cases for the University of Illinois reduced by half when it introduced disclosure. Only one patient sued in thirty-seven cases of preventable error. When medicine is participative, the patient is involved in the decisions, the responsibility is shared, and the blame game short-circuited.

The Example of Intravenous Injections

To be specific, we can consider a routine nursing task—administering an intravenous (IV) injection. This is a simple task but has the potential to cause harm. Sadly, the current practice is poor and many injections are done improperly; in one study, in 212 out of 430 injections, an error occurred.[40] Three of these mistakes were potentially severe; of the remainder, 29 percent were moderate and 19 percent were considered minor. The majority of problems occurred when giving rapid injections or in preparing the drug.

We can see how to prevent these errors by considering the processes the nurses use to prepare and give the injection. Both nurses and the hospital should consider intravenous injections as an invasive procedure. Nurses need sufficient time to perform the task; even on a busy ward, appropriate time should be allocated to the injection. Giving an intravenous injection should not be rushed nor be considered routine.

First, the nurse reads and considers the prescription. Only 3 percent of the errors were caused at this prescription stage. These errors could be reduced if the nurse consciously ensures that the prescription is clearly and unambiguously written and that she understands it. Clarification of any unclear instruction should be encouraged and considered standard procedure.

There are three types of preparation for an IV injection. The first two, a single-step preparation or a drug ready to be administered, have low risk. These can be performed by a trained nurse without particular concern, as significant risk has not been identified. We suggest, however, that the nurse routinely double checks both before and after the preparation. Multiple-step preparations are risky and give rise to 14 percent of the errors. This is unsurprising. What is surprising is that nurses with various levels of expertise are expected to mix drugs on the ward. Nurses preparing multiple-step injections should be specifically trained and certified for the procedure. We suggest that pharmacists prepare multiple step injections, because they are trained in this task and in procedures for quality control. Particular care is warranted for the transfer of information from the ward to the pharmacy.

The largest number of errors occurred during the process of injection. Rapid injections cause the largest number of errors (73 percent), intermittent infusions were less risky (9 percent), and no errors were noted for continuous infusions. The main problem appears to be administering the drugs too rapidly. A bolus dose should typically be given over a period of three to five minutes. Nurses should be made aware of the necessity to give slow IV doses and explicit training to time the injection could be implemented.

In this example, there were no errors in the identification of the patient. However, nurses could be trained to ask the patient's name before every injection. If the patient is unable to communicate, the nurse should check the name tag. Blame for an IV error does not rest with the individual nurse. The supervisor, medical staff, and organizational culture are all at fault if an error occurs. Staff should feel comfortable reporting errors and methods should be introduced to update the way the treatment is delivered.

SEVEN DEADLY MANAGEMENT DISEASES AND HOW TO FIX THEM

Dr. Deming described a number of management "diseases" that lead to reduced quality.[41] These are often characteristic of government organizations and particularly hospitals.

1. Lack of consistency of purpose—The purpose of the organization should be clear to all involved. The aim of a hospital is to help people heal. Doing harm is to be avoided by all staff, under all conditions. The aim is to improve the quality of the patients' experience and health. At the same time, these improvements should decrease the costs of care to the patient.

2. Emphasis on the short-term—Hospitals are concerned with short-term profitability and gains. Short-term considerations are obstructive. For example, hospital nutrition is poor because the hospital's aim is to deal with critical short-term conditions; so, it is assumed that nutrition does not matter—all the hospital needs to do for patients is "patch them up and send them home." By contrast, each stay in hospital could be a practical demonstration of nutritional excellence and disease prevention. A hospital's long-term goal should be continuous improvement, with the aim of providing an efficient, effective, and excellent service to their patients.

3. Evaluation by performance, merit rating, or annual review—Recent changes in hospital management to improve efficiency and cost effectiveness and to increase quality have resulted in the imposition of performance checks. Giving merit ratings or annual reviews of hospitals or hospital staff gives the appearance of monitoring quality, while it in reality prevents real improvement. In Dr. Deming's words, "Eliminate management by numbers, numerical goals. Substitute leadership."

4. Mobility of management—Moving management and senior staff may give the appearance of increasing expertise, but it means that the most expert managers are not used effectively. Staff need to be comfortable in their role and given time to gain experience. Gaining expertise takes time and is unlikely to be achieved in less than ten years' direct experience. "The aim of supervision should be to help people, machines, and gadgets to do a better job."

5. Running a hospital on visible measures—The central role of a hospital is for healing. Healing is not easily quantified or measured. Continuous improvement is not compatible with quotas.

6. Excessive medical costs—Hospital staff should use the facilities in their hospital with no special privileges or deals when they get sick. They should pay for their treatment in the same way as typical patients, receive the same treatment, and not have special insurance privileges. They would then know what it was like to be a patient in that hospital.

7. Excessive costs of warranty—Hospitals are currently hampered by excessive legal costs, resulting from low-quality service. Get rid of the lawyers who work for contingency fees. Let medical professionals work in a supportive environment, creating their own objectives for improved treatment standards and patient support. Replace lawyers with participative medicine.

Dr. Deming also described a number of lesser obstacles to achieving quality service. The first obstacle is neglect of long-range planning—that current medicine fails in this respect is clear from its emphasis on treatment rather than disease prevention. A similar limitation is the current reliance on technology to solve problems. Multimillion-dollar diagnostic systems and new cancer drugs costing $50,000 a year are no substitute for avoiding disease.

Dr. Deming suggested seeking successful examples to follow rather than developing solutions. In medical terms, a manager should find a doctor who does not get sued, a ward that does not get infections, a hospital with an excellent reputation, and then copy what they are doing. He could almost have been criticizing the current emphasis on so-called evidence-based medicine, the aim of which is supposedly to "prove" treatments using large-scale, randomized clinical trials without an underlying philosophy. In this approach, each treatment is tested individually, and scientific theory and models are belittled. There is no underlying intellectual theme, but rather a collection of experimental results.

Dr. Deming described a final obstacle—the "our problems are different" excuse. Medicine relies on this excuse to avoid facing reality. The management of medicine is no different from management of other complex organizations and high technology systems.

CHAPTER 4

A Look at Hospital-Acquired Infections

*"The very first requirement in a hospital
is that it should do the sick no harm."*
—FLORENCE NIGHTINGALE (1820–1910)

When you need to go into a hospital, you hope to expect to return healthy. But one in twenty inpatients will return with a hospital-acquired infection. Such infections are sometimes described as nosocomial. The United States has the most expensive health care in the world, and yet a decade ago, about half a million people suffered a hospital-derived infection each year, and 88,000 died from it; that's one person every six minutes, day and night.[1] The rate of hospital infection continues to grow and the culprit microorganisms have become increasingly resistant to antibiotics.[2]

The early success of antibiotics in the middle of the last century generated hubris in doctors. They thought that they had beaten infectious disease. Antibiotics and vaccination were technologies that appeared to be so effective that medicine had apparently triumphed. Any capable biologist could have told them that the microorganisms would simply adapt and evolve. There might be one or two successes, such as the eradication of smallpox, but the vast majority of microorganisms would hardly be affected. Old infections would develop defenses to accommodate and resist antibiotics at an exponentially increasing rate, and new diseases would emerge for which medicine had no effective response. It seems obvious in hindsight, but to the doctors, hubris replaced insight.

67

THE SICKEST PEOPLE IN CLOSE PROXIMITY

A modern hospital contains society's sickest people in close proximity. For this reason, a key feature is the need to prevent the spread of infections. Historically, some hospitals overcame the problem of infection by not admitting contagious patients. In 1219, when the Hospital of St. John, in Bridgewater, England, was formed, statutes were clear: lepers, pregnant women, infants, and patients with contagious disease were excluded. If they were allowed in by error, they were to be removed.[3] Difficult patients or the mentally ill were also unwelcome. Medieval English hospitals often discouraged admission of the sick.[4] Conversely, until recent decades, high death rates discouraged women from giving birth in a hospital. This was despite the early research showing that puerperal fever was an avoidable contagious disease.[5]

Hospital design has typically reflected the technology and scientific understanding of the day. The London Hospital, built in 1791, had its operating theaters on the top floor. The roof let in light to assist the surgeon, but this was not the real reason for its location. The top floor had large heavy doors that were closed before any operation started. In pre-anesthetic days, such doors served to muffle the screams of the patients. Perhaps the doors also functioned to keep patients in the hospital. Since hospital staff were needed to hold down and subdue the patients being operated on, other patients hearing the screams might otherwise take the opportunity to leave.

By the time the Johns Hopkins Hospital was built, in the late nineteenth century, sick patients were more welcome. An isolation ward was proposed to keep contagious or smelly patients apart.[6] Around the same time, the design and function of hospitals was beginning to be transformed by Florence Nightingale. In the 1920s, Asa Bacon, of Chicago's Presbyterian Hospital, proposed hospitals with all private rooms.[7] Bacon considered efficient hospitals should have rooms like hotel suites, with central heating and a private lavatory. Many modern hospitals do not achieve these levels of patient care.

By the 1990s, architects were expected to work with infection control professionals in the design of hospitals.[8] The recommendations for new hospitals were becoming more advanced. For example, new hospitals may use HEPA (high-efficiency particulate air) filters to lower the number of fungal spores in the atmosphere and lower the risk of aspergillosis, a particular problem with immunocompromised patients. HEPA filters can incorporate ultraviolet light to destroy bacteria, viruses, and fungal spores trapped by the filter media and provide protection against airborne disease transmission. Notably, HEPA and other air filters have been a mainstay of alternative medicine for decades. As with many buildings, the water supply and particularly drinking water in hospitals can be a source of legionella.[9] Hospitals should have filtered water free of such pathogens.

Tuberculosis (TB) is an excellent example of the problems with hospitals. A large hospital should have sealed rooms with negative pressure and frequent air changes for these patients. Approximately 9 million people worldwide develop active TB each year, and between 1 and 3 million die from the illness. However, perhaps 1 in 3 people have been infected but do not show symptoms.[10] That means around 1.7 billion people may have latent TB.[11] Whatever the actual numbers, many people become and remain infected with TB, long term, without having the illness or showing symptoms. Only about one in ten of those infected with TB will get the illness. Once symptoms appear, about half will die.

The reason that most people infected with TB do not get ill was stated clearly by Louis Pasteur on his deathbed: "The microbe is nothing, the terrain is everything." People get ill with TB when their immune system is compromised. This can be a result of inadequate nutrition, immunosuppressive drugs, substance abuse, or AIDS. In the old days, TB was treated in sanitaria, with sunlight and fresh air. This was a reasonable approach, as sunlight generates large amounts of protective vitamin D in the skin. Nutrition may play a large part in why so few with the latent infection become ill. Poor nutrition, particularly deficiency of vitamins C and D,[12] may lower host resistance allowing TB and other infections to take hold.

Make sure you are not susceptible to a hospital-acquired infection by taking orthomolecular levels of vitamins C and D_3. If the hospital staff tell you the nutrients will not work, remember that they are the people responsible for unnecessary hospital infections.

POOR MEDICAL HYGIENE

Before the germ theory of disease, medicine could be excused for lack of hygiene. It is difficult even to suggest that physicians could have noted the association with disease as dirt was ever present. Doctors of the eighteenth century did not know to wash their hands before surgery or between patients. Ignaz Semmelweis (1818–1865) tried to get doctors in obstetric clinics to wash their hands to prevent the spread of childbed fever. In 1847, Dr. Semmelweis was ignored when he discovered that lack of hygiene was killing women who were giving birth in the hospital. When doctors could be persuaded to wash their hands and conform to basic hygiene standards, death from sepsis fell from 22 percent to 3 percent.[13] Sadly, doctors in Dr. Semmelweis's time could not see the point of washing their hands and did not believe the evidence.

Some relatively recent doctors have displayed a similar disregard for hand washing. Even in the 1990s, rates of hand washing were low and there was a need for education in essential hygiene.[14] Doctors did not appear to understand the need for basic hand washing.[15] During twenty-one hours of ward rounds, consultants were reported to wash their hands only twice.[16] In one study, 939 patient contacts were observed and the hand-washing rates both before (12.4 percent) and after (10.6 percent) patient contacts were measured.[17] Medical staff were more diligent when they knew they were being watched: when openly observed, rates increased, leveling out at 32.7 percent (before) and 33.3 percent (after). Following performance feedback, these rates increased to 68.3 percent (before) and 64.8 percent (after). Seven weeks after the study, medical staff were observed covertly again. Hand-washing rates were then 54.6 percent before and 54.9 percent after patient contact. So, when medical staff are in an environment that expects and acknowledges the importance of hygiene, they can adopt more reasonable practices.

When doctors are asked about hand washing, they thought they washed their hands 73 percent of the time. Direct observation indicated that their actual rate was only 9 percent.[18] Medical staff do not appreciate the consequences of not being diligent, even when the importance of hand washing is explained. When the *British Medical Journal* published an editorial on hand washing in 1999, the responses were startling. Dr. Andrew Weeks, a specialist in obstetrics and gynecology, explained why he did not wash his hands between patient contacts, saying "I have never seen any convincing evidence that hand washing between each patient contact reduces infection rates."[19] Despite working in the same area of medicine as Dr. Semmelweis, he explained that with sixty touch contacts with patients each day, there was simply insufficient time for all this hand washing. Dr.

Weeks' argument echoes back down the decades, reminiscent of early doctors' responses to Dr. Semmelweis.

Dr. S. Kesavan, a senior resident physician, provided practical reasons for lack of hand washing, citing the lack of facilities for hand washing in hospitals.[20] Nurses were concerned about possible damage to their skin.[21] A letter from Dr. Robert MacDermott, another senior registrar in obstetrics and gynecology, suggested that dermatitis was a possible consequence of repeated hand washing.[22] He noted the use of gloves as protection and suggested that appropriate solutions for hand washing should be provided. This is unlikely to be sufficient, as even the uniform of the hospital doctor is dangerous. Dr. Varghese, a cardiothoracic surgeon, noted that stethoscopes[23] and white coats[24] spread disease in hospitals.

In the 1990s, it seems, hospitals were poorly managed with insufficient attention to basic hygiene. Kesavan and colleagues investigated the adequacy of hand washing facilities at 264 sinks on nineteen elderly care wards in seven hospitals in the United Kingdom.[25] There were numerous deficiencies: many sinks were inaccessible, badly placed, or blocked by ward equipment; ward sinks often did not have soap, antiseptic agent, or hand cream. Dr. Kesavan recommended the implementation of a standard checklist for hospital hand-washing facilities. Given this lack of management, it is hardly surprising that hospitals develop widespread antibiotic-resistant diseases.

Hospital staff are little more hygienic than members of the public. Paul Hateley, lead nurse for infection control at the Royal Hospitals, London, and P.A. Jurnaa, consultant microbiologist at Great Ormond Street Hospital, performed an observational study and reported that 59 of 100 male and 83 of 100 female health-care workers washed their hands after using the toilet. For comparison, they observed members of the public and found that 34 of 100 male and 56 of 100 female members of the public washed their hands after using a toilet in a railway station. Hateley and Jurnaa suggested that improvements in hospitals would be difficult, without changes in the wider community. However, we consider this special pleading—hospital staff have a particular and crucial need for such hygiene methods.

The above accounts concerned hospitals in the 1990s. It is likely that hospitals will use the age-old defense of medical progress. "Yes, in the bad old days of the 1980s and 1990s, standards were unacceptable. However, since that time progress has been made. We have improved hospital management. There are alcohol dispensers at the bottom of all our patients beds. Medical staff are trained in hygiene, and encouraged to wash their hands between patients . . ." And so on. However, a patient going into hospital is still far too likely to catch an antibiotic-resistant infection. Rather than improving, things seem to be getting worse.

The lack of care with even routine techniques can lead to infection. Each year, almost a million needle-stick injuries are reported in U.S. hospitals. Underreporting could mean the true incidence is nearer three million events. Data from the University of Virginia puts this into context.[26] In teaching hospitals, there was an average of thirty-three reported wounds per 100 beds; in other hospitals, the rate was sixteen per 100 beds. Yet, these are certified medical professionals—phlebotomists, nurses, and doctors—in high-technology environments.

FLORENCE NIGHTINGALE: A HERETICAL VIEW

The problem of hospital-acquired infections is not a new one. The *British Medical Journal* did a cover story to honor Florence Nightingale (1820–1910), who was perhaps the first media-created celebrity.[27] The widely supported choice of "the lady of the lamp" as medical heroine remains controversial. Nightingale gained fame and acceptance partly because of her ability as a self-publicist and partly because she was a bureaucrat. One biographer suggests that Nightingale was not even an efficient administrator but rather a power-hungry and manipulative person.[28] More moderate critics have pointed out that many of her achievements are mythical and a creation of the popular press.[29] Despite these claims, Florence Nightingale remains one of the most important historical figures in health care.

Nightingale was brilliant at self-promotion but rather a poor nurse. Her own sister, Parthenope, said of Florence, "She was a shocking nurse."[30] Nightingale was from a wealthy and well-respected family and her skills as a ruthless politician and administrator were respected by the establishment. Her popular support influenced contemporary politics. Perhaps this is unsurprising, as politicians and managers are prone to support people who place administration at the center of a problem. One of Nightingale's main contributions to hospital design was to discourage private rooms or multiple bays, which did not allow nurses to view all the patients at once.[31] She believed that the benefits of staff efficiency and increased monitoring in large multi-occupancy wards outweighed the need for individual privacy.

Guided by Florence Nightingale, the Victorian and later medical establishments built their hospitals and staffed them with nurses trained to her requirements. One common criticism is that Nightingale supported the miasma theory of infection. "Quarantine is a complete failure" is one quote from this famous lady.[32] She held on to the idea that disease was caused by smell long after the germ theory of disease was established in 1858 by Louis Pasteur. However, Nightingale's opinion later in life is not clear; some contend that her support of sterilization, antisepsis, and asepsis show she later gained an understanding of the germ theory and its implications.

Fortunately, avoiding bad smells has the side effect of preventing the spread of germs. Cleaning and good ventilation are common to both. The miasma theory led inadvertently to a massive reduction in infectious disease. In London, avoidance of bad smells led Sir Joseph Bazalgette (1819–1891) to develop modern sewers, preventing cholera and other water-borne disease. The world followed Bazalgette's initiative, leading to perhaps the greatest disease reduction in history.

Nightingale's influence on hospital design was largely determined by her advocating the invalid miasma theory of disease. In 1853, Nightingale visited the new Lariboisière Hospital in Paris and witnessed the design of the wards.[33] The new hospital had wards constructed on a pavilion plan. Since the miasma theory explained that disease arose in confined or dirty spaces, large rooms full of fresh air would prevent smells and the resulting disease and illness. The new wards admitted fresh air and light; long open corridors between the wards allowed the miasmas to disperse.

As late as 1898, Florence Nightingale's influential book *Notes on Nursing: What It Is, And What It Is Not*[34] concentrated on fresh air for cleanliness. She believed scarlet fever, measles, smallpox, and other infections were caused by houses being built over drains, from which odors could escape and sicken the inhabitants.[35] With this background, the emphasis of cleanliness, ventilation, and sunlight in the design of hospitals is understandable.

One substantial benefit arose from the potential for sunlight to increase vitamin D production and improve the health of patients. When exposed to the sun, people manufacture vitamin D_3 in their skin. Sunlight can also kill microorganisms. The large room volume and ventilation would have helped disperse airborne infections. Nightingale believed the lowered mortality in the Lariboisière hospital confirmed the miasma theory. For decades, the design of hospitals followed the Nightingale approach.

Nightingale's beliefs yielded improvement in hygiene as a side effect: cleaning, a way of removing the cause of smells, also removes germs. The result was reduced transmission of disease. Unfortunately, ideas with serendipitous side benefits are not ideal foundations for designing hospitals, health management, or training nurses.

At War

During the Crimean War (1853–1856), the British Government allowed Florence Nightingale to take thirty-eight nurses to help injured soldiers. The need was urgent—the Crimean War reportedly had four times as many deaths resulting from inadequate medical care than from battle. At first, Nightingale and her nurses had little influence on the death rate, as they ignored the need for sanitation.

Nightingale's Scutari hospital was not close to the battlefront in the Crimea, but rather 300–400 miles away in Istanbul. A wounded soldier needed to survive a long sea journey in order to reach the hospital. Injured soldiers would arrive with infected and blackened wounds. Often, they were infested with maggots, although, considering the action of maggots in cleaning wounds, these soldiers may have been relatively fortunate. If the soldier survived the journey, his chance of survival at Scutari was lower than if he had been too sick to transport.[36] In the first winter, 5,000 of 12,000 soldiers reaching the hospital died. After surviving the journey to Scutari, patients had a 42 percent chance of dying. Each nurse was responsible for at least eighty-four patients, so patients could rarely have received individual attention.

This was a perfect environment for administration and sanitation to have a large effect on survival. Nightingale and her nurses eventually cut the death rate from 427 per thousand to 22 per thousand. However, such a result was possible because of preexisting poor conditions at Scutari. Under such conditions, any improvements in cleaning, sanitation, and hygiene would be expected to lower the death rate.

It is often not reported that Nightingale ignored government commissioners' requests that she should first clean the wards and flush out the drains beneath the wards. She regarded them as interfering government busybodies. Men were dying—she did not have time to waste on cleaning sewers! However, the commissioners were right. Death rates were high in the hospitals, and Nightingale's hospital had the highest rates. The Royal commission covered up these failings of the national hero. Nightingale learned the lesson, however, and would later press consistently for light, clean hospitals, with excellent ventilation.

Interestingly, Nightingale might have cleaned the hospital after being scolded by another woman. Miranda Stuart (1795–1865), or perhaps her real name was Margaret Ann Bulkley,[37] masqueraded as a man so she could train and eventually become a qualified and successful doctor. In so doing, her alter ego, "Dr. James Barry," unofficially became the first British woman to be medically qualified. Dr. Barry heard of the squalor and high death rate at the Nightingale hospital and went over to see for herself. She eventually confronted Nightingale and gave what Nightingale described as the worst scolding of her life, while sitting, literally, on a high horse. While the content of this scolding is not fully established, some suggest that Dr. Barry was explaining the need for hygiene. Sanitation was certainly high on Dr. Barry's list of priorities.[38] Whatever the reason, the hospital's windows were opened and drains were cleaned out. In one week, 215 handcarts of muck were removed, the sewers were flushed, and the bodies of two horses, a cow, and four dogs were buried.[39]

MOTHER SEACOLE

If you could ask your ancestors whether their family doctor was female, you would get few positive answers and some strange looks. Furthermore, women physicians who did practice were usually graduates of homeopathic and naturopathic schools. Today, we tend to be unaware of this, because we are not told. Drug-centered physicians like to parade Elizabeth Blackwell's 1849 graduation, from Geneva Medical College, as heralding the first female doctor of "modern medicine" in the U.S. The educational and charitable works of Dr. Blackwell are well recorded. But pharmaceutically biased history has slipped quietly by the real story: nineteenth-century medical women had their roots and practices in herbal, hygienic, and nutritional therapies.

Naturopathy, a system of natural therapies that acknowledges and influences the innate healing potential of the body, is becoming increasingly popular as the limitations in modern medicine become apparent. The philosophical basis of naturopathy is similar to that of nursing. Naturopathy originated in the early history of medicine, with Hippocrates and others. Galen and Greek ideas dominated medicine for over a thousand years. Gradually, harmful remedies were introduced, such as bleeding, mercury, and purging. These are in direct contrast to the safer methods of natural medicine, which are closer to those of Hippocrates. Once the cause of the illness is found, the aim is to treat the whole patient holistically. Preventive medicine and education are central to the naturopathic approach.

Naturopathy was popular in the Victorian era, re-emerging in the time of Florence Nightingale.[40] In Nightingale's words, nursing was "the proper use of fresh air, light, warmth, cleanliness, quiet, and proper selection and administration of diet." Her approach to nursing was similar to that of a naturopath. Unfortunately, modern hospitals have strayed far from this emphasis on nutrition and support for the healing process.

Mary Seacole provided natural medical care during the Crimean War and was, in a way, a competitor to Nightingale. However, Seacole had several disadvantages: she was black and, though caring and competent, she typically dressed like a gypsy. Unlike Nightingale, Seacole did not have an influential family, with all the implied advantages. Moreover, she did not provide assistance by managing a hospital hundreds of miles from the battlefield: she was often on the front line, under fire, taking bandages and fluids to the injured.

Mary Seacole was born in Jamaica in 1805 and died of apoplexy (stroke) in London in 1881. Mother Seacole, as she became known, was famous for her work in the Crimean War. However, the designation "nurse" does not really suit Mary Seacole, who described herself as a "doctress." The word *doctress* has no modern meaning, but suggests a female doctor at a time when the profession was uniformly male. Seacole believed she was acting more like an unlicensed doctor than a contemporary nurse. Her unconventional healing was often, however, more effective than the best contemporaneous medicine had to offer.

Patients who wanted to survive and return to health would have been well advised to opt for Mother Seacole's help, rather than take the long sea passage to Scutari and risk the hospital. Seacole was operating in a world before the licensing of physicians and surgeons was fully implemented. In the 1850s, just before the extension of medical licensing in the U.K., Seacole's role was that of healer, herbalist, and battlefield surgeon. She had learned folk medicine and herbalism from her mother, who ran a Jamaican boarding house for disabled sailors and soldiers. When she became aware of the limited medical support for soldiers fighting in the Crimea, she moved to London and approached the War Office to offer help. In her words, this was "in blissful ignorance of the labor and time I was throwing away."[41] The salaried representatives of the government laughed at her application; the establishment has rarely had a reputation for open-minded thinking.

Despite her application and experience, Mary Seacole was not included in plans for the Crimea. She was, however, very determined and found her own funding to travel to the battlefield as an independent practitioner. Arriving at Scutari with a letter of introduction from a doctor, she was asked to wait to see Florence Nightingale, as Nightingale's time was too valuable to waste. After their meeting, Seacole was allowed to sleep in the washerwomen's quarters, before moving to the front line. It was a miserable vocation.

Mother Seacole's Medicine

By the end of the war, in early 1856, Mary Seacole had overextended her resources in providing treatment to the soldiers. Returning to London, her friends, who were also back from the war, held a concert for her benefit. In Victorian times, Seacole's medical work was acknowledged alongside that of Florence Nightingale. Like Nightingale, Seacole was an excellent self-publicist, and her book *Wonderful Adventures of Mrs. Seacole in Many Lands,* published in 1857, was well received. Her efforts were subsequently forgotten for nearly a century.

Recently, Seacole's work has been recognized again, and she is now seen as a brave black woman who succeeded in a Victorian world of racial and gender prejudice. Arguably, Seacole had more relevant experience with infectious diseases than most practicing doctors. In a Central American cholera epidemic in 1851, Seacole had treated the rich and, like a medical Robin Hood, used the profits to minister to the poor. Her first patient survived, enhancing her reputation and number of patients. She avoided using opium, but used the then conventional approaches, based on lead and mercury. More holistically, she employed a drink of cinnamon boiled in water; cinnamon is a known antibiotic.[42] With hindsight, we suspect that Seacole's success arose from her holistic approach of rehydration, infection control, and natural antibiotics, rather than the use of heavy metals. Notably, she varied her treatment according to the individual patient. Seacole's practical experience and the medical tradition of her people accommodated the reality of contagion, while Western medicine took many years to accept and act on the germ theory.

A poem called "A Stir for Seacole" was published in 1856, in praise of Mary Seacole:

The sick and sorry can tell the story
Of her nursing and dosing deeds,
Regimental M.D. never worked as she
In helping sick men's needs.

HOSPITALS AND "SUPER-BUGS"

Recently, hospitals have again become known as centers of disease transmission of "super-bugs" that are resistant to antibiotics. A typical hospital environment is contaminated with MRSA (methicillin-resistant *Staphylococcus aureus*),[43] VRE (vancomycin-resistant enterococci),[44] *Clostridium difficile*,[45] and so on. Despite hospitals being designed to prevent transmission, patients quite rightly perceive them as sources of infection.

Partly, this reflects a laissez-faire attitude to infectious disease, following the introduction of antibiotics. Doctors and other health professionals overused antibiotics for years, promoting resistant organisms. According to the U.S. Centers for Disease Control and Prevention (CDC), antibiotic resistance "can cause significant danger and suffering for people who have common infections that once were easily treatable with antibiotics.... Some resistant infections can cause death."[46]

In addition, in the 1950s, the Food and Drug Administration (FDA) allowed antibiotics as animal growth promoters. This widespread use meant people were consuming antibiotics in their food. Decades after the mechanisms of antibiotic resistance were identified and appreciated, their misuse continues even today. Unfortunately and predictably, discovery and development of new antibiotics has lagged behind the rapid rise in resistance.[47] We are all at risk from this indiscriminate use of antibiotics.

Each year, over 3 million pounds of antibiotics are reportedly used in the U.S. medical system: enough to give every person in the country a teaspoonful of pure drug.[48] About half the patients with upper respiratory tract infections, such as the common cold, will be prescribed antibiotics. However, the majority of these infections are caused by viruses, against which antibiotics are ineffective. About 20 million of the 50 million prescriptions for antibiotics were unsuitable. In addition, each year, a staggering 25 million pounds of antibiotics are administered to farm animals, almost ten times the amounts used for humans. Mostly, these are given in an attempt to prevent illness or increase growth rates. Seepage from farms spreads low concentrations of antibiotics through our waterways and food. This misuse increases antibiotic resistance in organisms that cause human disease.[49]

In 2008, the CDC released the first report ever done on adverse reactions to antibiotics in the United States.[50] This is startling because antibiotics have been widely used since the 1940s. Why has it taken the CDC so long to report on the side effects of these drugs? It is now apparent that an undeserved presumption of safety has existed for decades.

Antibiotics can put you in the emergency room. Common antibiotics, the ones most frequently prescribed and regarded as safest, cause nearly half of such emergencies. Partly, their widespread use produces an increased number of adverse events. Incredibly enough, people in the prime of life, not babies, are especially at risk: people 15–44 years old accounted for 41.2 percent of emergency department visits; infants only accounted for 6.3 percent.[51] They also found that nearly 80 percent of antibiotic-caused adverse events were allergic reactions. Overdoses and mistakes, by patients and by physicians, make up the rest.

Allergic reactions to antibiotics can be serious, including life-threatening anaphylactic shock, a system-wide reaction. Anaphylactic shock is the most severe form of reaction and can cause death in minutes, if untreated. A search of the U.S. National Library of Medicine's "Medline" database for "antibiotic allergic reaction" generates over 10,000 scientific or medical papers. A search for "antibiotic anaphylactic shock" brings up over 1,100. Many papers on this severe danger were published before 1960.[52] Since that time, adverse reactions have accumulated, and one might wonder why the CDC took so long to investigate the problem.

Antibiotic resistance and allergic reactions continue to be major public health issues. Both dangers are directly related to the large amount of antibiotics we consume or feed to animals. One way to improve the situation would be to use antibiotics less often.

ALTERNATIVES TO ANTIBIOTICS

Alternative, non-drug treatments can be an answer to the problem of prevention and treatment of infection. Robert F. Cathcart, M.D., and several other doctors have independently reported that massive doses of vitamin C substantially lower the effective dose of antibiotics or eliminates their need. Vitamin C also specifically counters allergic reactions. According to Dr. Cathcart, "Patients seemed not to develop their first allergic reaction to penicillin when they had taken bowel tolerance vitamin C for several doses. Among the several thousand patients given penicillin, two cases of brief rash were seen in patients who had taken their first dose of penicillin along with their first dose of vitamin C. . . . Many patients find the effect of ascorbate [vitamin C] more satisfactory than immunizations or antihistamines and decongestants."[53]

Back in the 1940s and 1950s, physicians such as William J. McCormick, M.D., and Frederick R. Klenner, M.D., found that high doses of vitamin C can be safely and effectively used to treat infection, allergy, and shock.[54] The intakes of vitamin C employed in such therapy were far in excess of the commonly touted 1 gram (1,000 mg) "megadose" for treating colds. The initial oral intakes are as much as 5–10 grams every half hour, tailing off as symptoms subside or the beginnings of a laxative effect is apparent. This takes a little practice. Either the person takes too much too quickly, causing diarrhea, or too little, with no effect. In the words of Dr. McCormick, an early pioneer, "When thus administered, the effect in acute infectious processes is favorably comparable to that of the sulfonamides or the mycelial antibiotics, but with the great advantage of complete freedom from toxic or allergic reactions."[55] In other words, massive intakes of vitamin C can be more effective and safer than antibiotics.

While drug-oriented conventional medicine ignores the potential for nutrition in prevention and treatment, some other direct methods of infection control continue. Even today, hand washing is a primary preventive measure for preventing the spread of hospital infections. Check that your doctors and nurses wash their hands. (Yes, you have to be certain.) Rubber gloves are not always used, and they are not enough, even when they are used. Hand washing should be done before and, preferably, following a patient's examination. Ceilings and walls are not common sources of patient infection, unless they are damp or damaged. However, the walls,

The Strange Case of Vitamin C

The first physician to use massive doses of vitamin C to treat disease was Dr. Frederick R. Klenner (1907–1984), beginning back in the early 1940s. "Vitamin C is the safest substance available to the physician" was his credo. Dr. Klenner claimed to consistently cure chicken pox, measles, mumps, tetanus, and polio with huge doses of the vitamin, as much as 300,000 milligrams (mg) per day. Generally, he gave 350–700 mg per kilogram of body weight per day. Dr. Klenner emphasized that small amounts do not work: "If you want results, use adequate ascorbic acid."

Born in Pennsylvania, Dr. Klenner received his medical degree from Duke University in 1936, followed by three years of postgraduate training specializing in diseases of the chest. In the mid-1940s, he reported successful treatment of forty-one cases of viral pneumonia with vitamin C. Dr. Klenner's doses were enormous, continuous, and symptom-driven. The sicker the patient, the higher the dose. "When proper amounts are used, it will destroy all virus organisms," he said. "Don't expect control of a virus with 100 to 400 mg of C." Today, corporate medicine considers a single gram of vitamin C a high dose. Showing that a gram of vitamin C will not cure a cold is irrelevant; Drs. Klenner, Cathcart, and Levy reported effects with doses 100 times larger. Strangely, the reports of these physicians for massive intakes of vitamin C are not refuted or even tested in later clinical trials. Decades later, we still await scientific testing of these clinical observations.

floor, and air in hospitals may become contaminated. The floors harbor mostly skin organisms.[56] Cleanliness and ventilation in hospitals remain the primary way of preventing infection.

BE VIGILANT

A patient entering the hospital needs to be vigilant about hygiene, which is often easier said than done. We say again: you cannot rely on doctors having washed their hands before examination or treatment. So, if you do not see the doctor or nurse washing their hands, and are feeling sufficiently daring, remind them. Try to be courteous and respectful, but do not expect willing cooperation. However, if you have any concerns about your own immunity—for example, if you have had chemotherapy or are a transplant patient—forget about politeness and demand that they wash their hands.

More importantly, ensure that your immune system is reinforced with good nutrition before, during, and after your hospital stay. In particular, make sure you have sufficient vitamin D_3 (5,000 units a day) and vitamin C. With vitamin C, try to achieve constant level of at least 50 percent of your bowel tolerance by taking supplements every four to six hours if possible. You may expect that the hospital will not like the supplements.

Later in this book, we will offer practical steps you can take to protect yourself from infection if you have to stay in the hospital.

CHAPTER 5

Psychiatry and the Limits of Modern Medicine

"Most men are within a finger's breadth of being mad."
—Diogenes the Cynic (404–323 BCE)

Looking back in time, the treatment of psychiatric patients seems less than sane and has been consistently awful. Psychiatric hospitals and treatment centers have not been known for their ability to cure patients; most of those that come into their care are managed rather than cured. In the eighteenth century, mental hospitals, such as Bethlem Royal Hospital (also known as Bedlam), in London, supplemented their funding by allowing the public to view the lunatics. The conditions were frightful. Patient care was largely restraint: uncooperative patients were manacled and chained to the wall. The noise alone was reported to be enough to drive a person insane. Some lucky patients were permitted to leave and beg in the streets in an effort to survive. It is humbling to remember that the beggars in modern city streets are often also mentally ill. Some still prefer the streets to psychiatry.

Schizophrenia remains one of the most serious chronic diseases, attacking 1 to 2 percent of the population. Fifty years ago, patients suffering from schizophrenia occupied half of all the mental hospital beds and one-quarter of all hospital beds. Today, most of the mental hospitals have shut down but they have not disappeared. The mental hospitals were closed, shrunk in size, or incorporated into wards in general hospitals. By refusing to accept patients, and by discharging them before they are ready for independent living, they converted the wider community into the new mental hospitals. About half of the homeless people on our streets are schizophrenics, many of whom have been treated in mental hospitals or psychiatric wards, placed on tranquilizers, and then discharged to fend for themselves in a hostile world.

Formerly, mental patients were treated in inadequate hospitals, which provided shelter, food, and some medical care. Patients were protected from society and, in turn, society was protected from the more violent aggressive psychotics. The patients, aggressive or not, had little personal freedom. Today, the modern mental hospital is the street: rundown hotels, nursing homes, foster homes, and so on deal with the mentally ill. They provide tranquilizers for some, but little food or shelter. There is no longer protection for patients or for society. The patients implicitly have freedom to be sick, to roam, and to refuse medication. They also prey upon and are preyed upon by others. Life for schizophrenics is a severe struggle, because of inadequate treatment and support.

Early treatments, such as electroconvulsive therapy (ECT) and insulin coma, had been introduced with the idea that schizophrenia and other mental disorders were biochemical in nature. These treatments apparently increased the recovery rate slightly, though the benefits were temporary. Mental diseases are typically long term, more like diabetes than appendicitis, and need lasting programs of treatment that are relatively free of side effects.

Modern drugs, primarily the major tranquilizers, are helpful in ameliorating the symptoms of the disease, but these antipsychotics cannot and do not lead to recovery. Psychiatric chemotherapy does little good and leaves unfortunate patients with a dismal choice: they can decline the drugs and remain naturally psychotic or they can opt to suffer a drug-induced disease called tranquilizer psychosis. Antipsychotic drugs have severe side effects that increase with time and can cause permanent neurological disability.

The end results for typical schizophrenics are the same—they do not recover. The recovery rate today is under 15 percent, which is apparently only one-third of the recovery rate achieved in 1850. The street schizophrenics today are no better off than they were in the mental hospitals of the 1950s. In those days, they suffered from psychiatric ignorance and social rejection. Today, they suffer from psychiatric refusal to embrace nutritional therapy. Dietary treatment provides patients with a choice that can enable them to become normal and stay well.

THE STIGMA OF MENTAL ILLNESS

Even today, mental illness is considered somehow shameful by many. Some have considered schizophrenia to be a socially constructed illness, a sane response to an insane world. While people with eccentric behavior may be misdiagnosed, mental illness can strike anyone and is clearly a physical disease. We are all potential patients and it is easy to induce psychosis. Shortage of vitamin B_3 will consistently bring about psychosis in otherwise normal, mentally strong people. Lack of a small amount of this single nutrient can bring on schizophrenia or related psychosis. That disturbed beggar may be someone with who was unfortunate enough to have a higher-than-typical need for vitamin B_3 and a teenager's taste for a junk food diet. People with psychosis are not weak, pathetic people—they simply have an illness that could under the right circumstances affect anyone.

Governments and managers running psychiatric hospitals have been concerned about the stigma associated with institutionalism. One approach was to relocate psychiatric hospitals away from centers of population. In Saskatchewan, the two large hospitals were at least seventy-five miles away from Saskatoon and Regina, the two main cities. The names were changed and they were no longer called asylums, as this indicated insanity. In Saskatchewan, they were often named after the location, which did not help, since you cannot flee from stigma by giving it a pretty name.

At the University Hospital to which Dr. Hoffer moved in 1954, the psychiatric ward was not named—it was simply called "5DE" for its two wards, 5D and 5E. Locally, 5DE soon had the same stigma as the word *asylum*. When Dr. Saul was a student at the Canberra Hospital, Australia, the corresponding name was "R-Wing." Recovery of patients from these wards might have de-stigmatized them, but that that did not happen. Changing the name did not fool the public.

Back in the nineteenth century, British psychiatrist John Conolly was aware of the ease with which a person could be considered mentally ill and the difficulty of reversing the diagnosis. He said, "Let no one imagine that even now it is impossible or difficult to effect the seclusion of an eccentric man or easy for him when once confined to regain his liberty."[1] More recently, in 1970, American psychologist David Rosenhan conducted an experiment to demonstrate that the problem continues.[2] Eight normal people, including psychologists and psychiatrists, presented themselves at psychiatric clinics claiming to hear unclear voices, including the word "thud." They were otherwise to act normally. If admitted, they were to explain they felt fine and the voices had stopped. Seven were diagnosed as schizophrenic and the last as manic depressive. Once in the hospital, getting out was difficult. The other patients identified them as sane, but they were unable to convince the doctors. They would not be released until they admitted they were ill and took antipsychotic medication. Today, things are different—the experimenters would probably be encouraged to leave the hospital as soon as they had been sufficiently tranquilized.

Of course, corporate medicine used the same old defense. They updated their methods and claimed that normal people could no longer be classified as insane. The introduction of a new diagnostic manual of psychiatric disorders (the American Psychiatric Association's *Diagnostic and Statistical Manual of Mental Disorders* or DSM-3) was supposed to prevent such problems. Indeed, Dr. Robert Spitzer, one of the leading psychiatrists, suggested that Rosenhan's study was pseudoscience.[3] With the new methods Dr. Spitzer announced, "that experiment could never be successfully repeated. Not in this day and age."

Psychologist Lauren Slater was writing a book on great psychological experiments and covered Rosenhan's study.[4] Much to her husband's chagrin, Slater decided to try to repeat the test in an up-to-date hospital. She visited emergency rooms for a psychiatric assessment after saying she heard the word "thud." In nine visits, she was consistently diagnosed as suffering depression with psychosis and prescribed antipsychotics. In Slater's words, "I am prescribed a total of twenty-five antipsychotics and sixty antidepressants. At no point does an interview last longer than twelve-and-a-half minutes, although at most places I needed to wait an average of two-and-a-half hours in the waiting room."

Psychiatry is not a science—it is based on subjective observation of behavior. Despite psychosis being a clear neurological condition, when a person is diagnosed as mentally ill or psychotic there is no hard evidence to support the assertion. There are no officially recognized biochemical measurements or other changes in the person's physiology. Psychiatrists note that a patient is behaving strangely or providing supposedly irrational responses to questions. The standard symptoms are things like the person reports hearing voices. Sometimes, the psychiatrist will try to support his contention with the results of magnetic resonance imaging (MRI) or positron emission tomography (PET) scans that show changes in the brain of diagnosed individuals. However, there are many environmental influences and medical interventions that alter brain images and the results may not be specific to the diagnosis. Psychiatrists should realize their discipline is not scientific and would be well advised to show a little humility.

LACK OF TREATMENT CHOICE

When no safe treatment is available for a disease, and a physician claims to have found a safe and effective therapy, it is often rational to use the new treatment. Provided the new treatment is safe, this approach avoids toxicity and minimizes harm. However, doctors who are puzzled by the demands of so-called evidence-based medicine need to be weaned from an apparently uncontrollable addiction to prescribing drugs. This compulsion means they will recommend drugs even if the side effects outweigh possible benefits. Ill-informed doctors and patients like to use the latest and greatest medication, believing it may provide the breakthrough needed to cure a disease. This is a risky strategy as, when a drug first comes onto the market, its potential to cause adverse events or even death is unknown.

If all you have is a hammer, as the saying goes, everything looks like a nail. For example, if confronted with a disturbed, hyperactive, or aggressive child, along with the child's desperate parents, a modern child psychiatrist will tend to prescribe long-term, toxic drugs. Psychiatrists feel safe with this approach, which will not result in censure from the governing medical organizations. Modern medicine has forgotten that, before drugs became available, we used to treat children by methods that were safer and more rational for both child and society.

Early treatment paid attention to nutrition, food allergies, long-term health, and community support. Drug use was more circumspect and controlled. Specific drugs were available for known physical diseases, such as anticonvulsants for epilepsy. When Dr. Hoffer and others developed orthomolecular psychiatry and treated patients with supplements, it was safe and apparently effective for children.[5] Dr. Hoffer described the treatment of over 2,000 children under the age of fourteen: when nutritional medicine was used, few children needed powerful antipsychotic drugs. Nearly all the children recovered. Just like adults, children deserve interested and intelligent physicians.

Antipsychotic poisons are routinely given for most psychiatric diagnoses. Often, poisons that do not kill you will slow you down, make you sick, and act as a tranquilizer. Before sophisticated laboratory tests were developed to select antipsychotic drugs, a catatonic test was used. A catatonic person has a tendency to remain in a fixed, stuporous state for long periods. If a chemical given to an animal made it catatonic, it was probably a tranquillizing drug. Drug-induced catatonia is a superb controller of behavior—a person who can barely think, move, or talk will not exhibit unwanted behavior and will not need a straightjacket.

Unless catatonic behavior is the desired objective, a rational doctor would not force this state upon their patients. Of course, if a disruptive person is rendered catatonic, other people may benefit. However, it is not clear that being in a tranquilized state is better for the patient. Modern medicine has become so obsessed with drugs that it considers medication-induced catatonia preferable to difficult behavior. With misguided confidence, doctors assume that psychoses will never respond to simple vitamins and other natural compounds that are normally present in the body.

CORPORATE MEDICINE AND HERD BEHAVIOR

Dr. Hoffer attended the last meeting of the Huxley Institute of Biosocial Research (HIBR) in New York: he was president of the Institute and chaired the meeting. During the program, Dr. Allan Cott presented the case of a disturbed young boy, about eight years old, who refused to take his vitamin pills. Nevertheless, his mother was determined she would help him and had little sense of political correctness. Whenever she offered him the pills and he refused to take them, she would sit on him until he agreed! He recovered.

Dr. Cott left the stage and three other people marched on. First, was a short woman, about five feet four inches, who described the case from her point of view. Standing beside her was a tall, lanky, but healthy-looking young man, her son. He acknowledged what had happened and thanked her for having made him take the pills. The young woman standing beside him was his girlfriend. The standing ovation was astonishing—Dr. Cott had probably saved this family (and the New York social services) immense costs and suffering by prescribing a few pennies worth of vitamins. No drugs were used.

Dr. Hoffer began treating problem children about fifty years ago. The

---

Psychotherapy or Nutrition?

Dr. Allan Cott (1910–1993) gave up psychotherapy to specialize in the nutritional treatment of the mentally ill. He found that psychotherapy was ineffective in the early treatment of schizophrenia. He tried nutritional therapy and was sufficiently convinced to become an original member of the Committee on Therapy of the American Schizophrenia Association. According to Dr. Cott, "The patient with a biochemically disturbed brain is not capable of understanding or benefiting from the insights offered by conventional therapy."[6] He was a supporter of orthomolecular psychiatry and the use of niacin. However, he cautioned against patients self-medicating. "When you use niacin in such large doses, it acts more like a drug than a vitamin. That's why I don't think laymen should experiment with megavitamin therapy on their own. They should consult a physician first."

Dr. Cott also believed in the benefits of fasting. Books, even paperback best-sellers, can sometimes change lives. For many people, their introduction to therapeutic fasting came by way of Alan Cott's *Fasting: The Ultimate Diet* and *Fasting as a Way of Life*. When Dr. Saul first tried fasting as a self-treatment, he noticed that it was the best he'd ever felt while sick. Reading Dr. Cott's book set Dr. Saul on the path of learning about nutritional medicine.

---

recovery of the second child he treated with niacinamide (vitamin B_3), in 1960, made a lasting impression. This eight-year-old girl had been labeled retarded, a term that is no longer used, as it is considered humiliating. The girl in question was disturbed and restless; she was developing behavioral problems and was being prepared for special classes for the retarded. She had been adopted by her grandparents because her mother, who was pregnant, was in a chronic ward in a mental hospital. Dr. Hoffer saw a cute-looking little girl but, being inexperienced in children's illness, he could not make an accurate diagnosis. Rather than ignoring her problems, he suggested she be treated with a gram of niacinamide, three times a day after meals. Two years later, there had been no apparent change. Despite this, Dr. Hoffer encouraged them to continue the vitamin. Over the following two years, she blossomed and became normal. She completed her university education, became a teacher, and, a few years ago, she retired.

Doctors are currently trained to find such case studies unconvincing. Trained on the basis of statistical medicine, they neglect the importance of clinical observation. In this case, Dr. Hoffer had seen the girl twice in two years and, on each occasion, for only a few minutes. Others agreed the girl had made a recovery but suggested it was spontaneous ("just one of those things"). There was no shortage of explanations. Like the six blind-folded men who examined an elephant, each provided a different expla-nation of the recovery. Naturally, the consistent opinion was that it could not have been the vitamin.

However, Dr. Hoffer kept observing similar recoveries, together with the sad consequences of not treating these disturbed people properly. With the rise of statistical medicine, there is an unfortunate tendency for medics to consider only recent research results. This fits with the need for novel-ty as a source of patentable treatments for corporate medicine, but it means that results more than a few years old are often considered worth-less. It is rather like a physicist rejecting Isaac Newton and Albert Einstein as out of date, or a biologist rejecting Charles Darwin. Drug companies further exploit this idea and have taught both doctors and the public to look upon newer and more expensive drugs as better. This sad situation continues, in spite of consistent and accumulating evidence to the contrary.

Parents of disturbed children and relatives of the psychotic typically do not realize that tranquilizers make animals catatonic. These pills have nice packaging and are not labeled poisons with skull-and-crossbones, as they should be. Why would a learned profession blindly prescribe such drugs, with little supportive evidence? Perhaps doctors are simply over-obedient to supposed authority.[7] As described previously, in Professor Stanley Mil-gram's experiments, most subjects were found to comply with requests to torture others, when ordered to do so by an authority figure in a white coat. Throughout history, doctors were willing to poison and perform painful surgery without benefit of anesthetic, provided a medical author-ity deemed it current practice. In modern medicine, authorities are large-ly determined by the availability of finance and thus pharmaceutical companies are dominant players.

One day, medical historians may use antipsychotics as an example of barbaric treatment. They may be considered alongside chaining patients to the wall in the old Bedlam hospital. But today, herd behavior and is alive and well in doctors and other social animals. When Dr. Hoffer was

An Avalanche of Medical Misinformation

John Tierney has described the tendency of strange ideas in medicine to behave like avalanches.[8] Take the idea that fat in food is bad for a person's health. This idea gained popularity in the 1950s, when a diet researcher named Ancel Keys suggested that cholesterol in the diet causes heart attacks. (It does not.) He found a correlation between levels of fat consumption and rates of heart disease, and wrongly assumed that the first caused the second. However, to obtain the link, some of the available data was ignored. Keys cherry-picked the data, hiding an alternate explanation that should have discredited this idea from the start. In arguing for fat, Keys omitted the association between heart disease and sugar consumption. Most people are aware that high fat in our food comes from modern diets: high-fat, high-sugar processed foods now dominate supermarket shelves.

To their credit, the American Heart Association at first denied the link between fat and heart disease. However, by 1988, the Surgeon General was warning that ice cream was a public-health threat, similar to cigarettes. Unfortunately for this hypothesis, low-fat diets do not prevent heart disease. Indeed, Dr. Atkins' famous high-fat, low-carbohydrate diet, which restricts intake of sugars, has been shown to improve the profile of lipids in the blood and, arguably, prevents heart disease. As Tierney put it, "cascades are especially common in medicine." An influential person gets a silly idea, selects data to confirm the suggestion, and the cascade begins, rapidly turning into an unstoppable avalanche. Despite the lack of evidence, research funds were poured into attempts to relate dietary fat to cardiovascular disease for half a century. Other, more plausible explanations, such as sugar over-consumption and nutrient insufficiency, were not funded. As a result, people died.

These medical misinformation cascades lead to widespread errors, based on a mistaken consensus. Tierney continues, "Doctors take their cues from others, leading them to over-diagnose some faddish ailment (called bandwagon diseases) and over-prescribe certain treatment (like the tonsillectomies, once popular for children)." Unable to keep up with the volume of research, doctors look for guidance from experts or, at least, someone who sounds confident. The current fad for statin drugs builds on and maintains the cholesterol–heart disease hypothesis. It is rare for medicine to admit an error; it simply moves on and waits for patients to forget.

Doctors are driven by authorities who have no preferred access to information and no advantage in analyzing data. The authorities try to maintain the illusion of expertise in the received medical wisdom. They tend to report what they are supposed to believe rather than what the data indicate. This process of social conformity[9] is vividly described as groupthink.[10] In short, your doctor believes what he or she is taught and, as a result, people keep dying.

sixteen, he spent the summer herding about forty cattle to keep them from invading neighboring land. Among his charges was a cow that apparently thought the neighbor's grass *was* always greener. Back then, in the great drought and depression of the 1930s, this was a serious business. The neighbor's crop was valuable and the cow's behavior most unwelcome. At each opportunity, she would appoint herself lead-cow and head off toward the greener grass. Immediately, the other cattle would line up behind her and, like a Roman army unit, they would advance on the adjoining fields. Dr. Hoffer had a good horse and a dog to help, but could never teach that determined cow that she was not allowed to trample the neighbor's land.

Dr. Hoffer concluded that cattle were dumb and unteachable and did not even have the intelligence of a mouse. Of course, he was wrong, since he was judging them from a human point of view. The cows were presumably rewarded by good pasture when they strayed. However, herd behavior was impressed on his mind. It gave him great comfort to remember the herd when observing the behavior of doctors under the spell of corporate medicine.

PSYCHOTHERAPY OF LITTLE VALUE IN SCHIZOPHRENIA

Dr. Hoffer conducted early double-blind experiments to test the ability of niacin for treating schizophrenics. However, he soon found that schizophrenic patients were no longer being admitted to the psychiatric ward. There was resistance among the clinical staff to the study. They refused to allow their patients to be included, so they diagnosed them as suffering from depression, anxiety, or psychopathy. However, the patients relapsed after discharge, and on readmission the doctors were forced to make a more accurate diagnosis. Fortunately, the study ran for several years and the initial dearth of patients was followed by abundance.

Psychiatrists were aware that schizophrenics did not respond to psychotherapy. Schizophrenia is a physiological disease requiring direct treatment rather than discussion. Dr. Hoffer interviewed one patient after a resident had been treating her with psychotherapy for several months. During the therapy, she kept on looking over his shoulder into the corner of the ceiling. He asked what was she looking at and she replied that her sister, who lived in Edmonton, was in the top corner of the room, looking down at her. A few days later, Dr. Hoffer informed the resident that the patient was hallucinating and psychotic. The resident changed the diagnosis and sent her to the nearby mental hospital.

Today, psychiatrists are generally aware that psychotherapy alone is of little value, but they also know that drugs, although helpful, do not return schizophrenic patients to normality. If they have a patient that they really want to treat, they will diagnose them as bipolar (manic-depressive) or depressed, which most patients are. Note that the same patient may be diagnosed as bipolar or schizophrenic by different psychiatrists. With a bipolar diagnosis, they can prescribe lithium or antidepressants. However, psychiatrists do not want to treat some patients—those who are especially difficult, troublesome, or have a dislikable personality. In such cases, patients may be diagnosed as having a personality disorder. Narcissists and psychopaths are considered untreatable. In any event, the result is that patients who are schizophrenic, and who might respond to appropriate treatment, are drugged, ignored and banished to the streets of our large cities.

SHOCKING CHILDREN

In Australia, electroconvulsive shock treatment (ECT) has become popular for children under age four. ECT involves passing an electric current through the head of an anesthetized patient in order to induce a seizure. Usually, a muscle relaxant is also employed, as people have a tendency to fracture limbs and other bones, if restrained physically.[11]

The problem is sufficiently out of control and unethical that the media have begun to break ranks with corporate medicine. The *Herald Sun* (January 25, 2009), reported that "the use of ECT in the state of Victoria has tripled in the private health sector in the past six years." During 2007–2008, over 18,000 people were given ECT; 55 children younger than age four were treated. During 2008, 6,197 people were treated against their will. We have reasonable information on the long-term damaging effects of ECT in adults but not in children, whose brains are still maturing.

Dr. Hoffer treated some adult patients with ECT but never children. All of Dr. Hoffer's patients who got ECT were also treated with niacin, which has been found to protect brain tissue against nerve degeneration. Niacin also appears to decrease the memory loss caused by ECT. Dr. Hoffer first observed this effect in 1953, when a middle-aged woman came to see him in a local mental hospital, one month after her last ECT. She was disoriented, lost, confused, and unable to function; her accompanying husband was also unhappy, not knowing how to help her. Although Dr. Hoffer knew that no treatment had been shown to help, he gave her 1 gram of niacin, three times a day, after meals. He knew it was safe, had helped with other types of confusional psychoses, and would do no harm. One month later, the couple came back and both were happy: she was normal. In this woman's case, the old rule that this condition could not be helped appeared to be wrong.

Since then, Dr. Hoffer observed the same effect hundreds of times. He considered that any doctor who gives ECT without niacin is committing malpractice. ECT causes damage to the brain. Since there is no long-term evidence about its efficacy and safety for children, there is no rational reason for its use by Australian psychiatrists.

TREATMENT RATHER THAN CURE

Tommy Douglas, who Canadians chose as the "greatest Canadian of all time" in a national vote (2004), was Premier of Saskatchewan, the father of Canadian Medicare, and leader of the New Democratic Party. He was also a friend of Dr. Hoffer and saw the impact of poor treatment when Dr. Hoffer interned at a mental hospital in Saskatchewan. This was over fifty years ago and psychiatry was in terrible shape: there were no effective treatments and the main approach was incarceration. Still, medicine was quicker to adopt new ideas than the profession is today. Without Premier Douglas's energy, enthusiasm, and zeal to help the mentally ill, there would have been little psychiatric research in Saskatchewan. Under his leadership, Dr. Hoffer's group was allowed to conduct research freely, in spite of intense antagonism from the psychiatric establishment.

An impression of the atmosphere back then can be gleaned from the

Saskatchewan Hospital, which built new barns for its horses and other livestock while patients in the hospital remained in their inhuman prisons. A senior administrator in the Department of Health stated privately that it was more important to give adequate care to the livestock than the patients. When Premier Douglas left Saskatchewan, Dr. Hoffer's research quickly sailed into stormy seas.

When Dr. Hoffer was young and naïve, he had an excellent relationship with the pharmaceutical industry and its representatives. Corporate medicine had developed hormones; it had helped determine the structure of some vitamins and made them available. Drug companies such as Merck provided valuable information about these new vitamins in copious amounts and distributed it freely to anyone who was interested.

With the support of corporate medicine, Dr. Hoffer performed the first double-blind clinical nutrition trial in psychiatry. His trials on schizophrenic patients were done using vitamins (niacin and niacinamide) provided free by Merck. Merck deserves recognition for having helped discover that niacin (vitamin B_3) lowers cholesterol levels. Niacin, but not niacinamide, has the effect of returning blood lipids to a healthy profile more effectively than the overhyped statin drugs.[12] Inositol niacinate, the most common "no-flush" niacin, will also serve but is not as effective as niacin for lowering cholesterol. Both inositol hexaniacinate and niacinamide are as good as niacin for other conditions, such as psychoses, schizophrenia, and anxiety. However, they could not make the enormous profits now characteristic of the industry without patent protection.

Drug sales today are more dependent on promotion and advertising than they are on the merits and safety of the products. Corporate medicine depends upon "blockbuster drugs" that have some effect in relieving the symptoms of chronic disease. Their aim is treatment rather than cure. Treating a chronic disease produces a steady income stream. A cure, by contrast, might need to retail at more than $30,000 for it to be commercially interesting. People could question the necessity and cost of such a curative drug, but might willingly pay $50 a month for the rest of their life for symptom relief.

Common diseases such as arthritis, cardiovascular disease, and blood pressure disorders provide steady income. Illnesses that generate fear, such as cancer, can be highly profitable. People are willing to pay large sums and suffer the side effects from ineffective chemotherapy for even a slight chance of recovery. Corporate medicine does not put in the same effort to develop inexpensive drugs that are used only for a short period of time, like antibiotics, or drugs for rare illnesses, or for diseases of the Third World. This is not unethical: drug companies exist to make profits. The people who run corporate medicine have a legal obligation to maximize profits for their shareholders; they should not be expected to be altruistic.

The tragic irony is that, for many of these conditions, we already have natural treatments that can be more effective, free of side effects, and cheaper.

ANTIPSYCHOTIC DRUGS DO NOT CURE SCHIZOPHRENIA

Psychiatric patients do not like their medication, but neither would anyone else. In the short term, antipsychotics leave the patient barely able to think or communicate. Dry mouth, constipation, gaining weight, and skin disorders occur in the early stages of drug use. With continued use, especially with higher doses, patients often demonstrate a characteristic "thorazine shuffle." This slow, aimless stagger is a direct consequence of excess sedation with chlorpromazine, which also results in indifference to stimulation. With time, more severe and permanent adverse reactions start to appear. So, it is hardly surprising that some patients prefer the disease to typical antipsychotic medications.

All the major tranquilizer drugs used in psychiatry cause brain damage. The amount of the damage depends on the total dose accumulated. Thus, if a patient takes 100 milligrams each day of one of the older drugs for 1,000 days, the total dose is 100,000 mg or 100 grams. The total dose is found by multiplying the average daily dose by the number of days on that drug. Rather than tranquility, as the name suggests, these major tranquilizers cause misery.

Antipsychotic drugs are often worthless and cause more harm than benefit.[13] At common therapeutic doses, they take away a patient's ability to think and act. By increasing the dose, they can stop almost any thinking or behavior the therapist wants to stop by putting the patient out of action. This is not therapy—it is disabling people. Psychiatrists need to be more circumspect about using drugs known to be neurotoxic. These major tranquilizers may even permanently destroy a person's personality; the good aspects are removed with the bad. The drugs may relieve psychotic anxiety but they dull the personality, removing initiative, emotional reactivity, enthusiasm, sexual drive, alertness, and insight.

Antipsychotics do not cure schizophrenia. It may simply be that higher mental functions are more vulnerable and are impaired before the elementary functions of the brain, such as motor control. Loss of motor functioning is readily observed and is reported as a side effect. However, by the time motor controls are impaired, the brain's higher functions will also be damaged. As the dose and duration of medication increases, so does the atrophy of the cerebral cortex.[14] When a patient has been on antipsychotic drugs for some time, it can be difficult to tell whether degenerative changes in the brain are due to the illness or the drugs.

The widespread and somewhat indiscriminate use of these drugs is increasing. They have been used whenever it would suit someone to render a patient malleable and tranquil. This use is preparing the ground for millions of chronic schizophrenic and other patients to become more brain damaged. Note that schizophrenic patients have no choice: they may be forced to remain on the drugs, even if they know they are destroying their brains.

The increasing numbers mean that hundreds of thousands of people will be rendered helpless and in need of long-term care. It is not clear how corporate medicine is going to deal with the resulting brain-damaged schizophrenic patients. Even now, people are being taken from the mainstream of life, which passes them by. We are generating a permanent core of helpless people with little hope they will recover. Hospitals are freed from the large numbers of psychiatric patients that they fail to treat adequately. Dr. Hoffer estimated that nine out of ten of these patients could lead relatively normal productive lives.

PSYCHIATRIC DRUGS AND THE ABUSE OF POWER

In the past, mental hospitals harbored many of the abuses of modern medicine, as patients were assumed to be incapable of making rational decisions about their own health. With such patients, the hospital and doctors have complete authority and control. Even in ordinary hospitals, patients often lose power and choice over their bodies. With psychiatric patients, this process is taken to the extreme.

In the Middle Ages, lepers were declared dead to the world but alive to God.[15] The ceremony to proclaim them legally dead involved standing male patients in a grave and pouring soil on their heads. The afflicted person's possessions were transferred to their family and heirs, and the lepers were sent to isolated colonies and, if they were lucky, were left food and drink. Often, they had to fend for themselves or, perhaps, to risk being burnt to death. This removal of legal rights and isolation has parallels with modern-day psychiatric patients. However, with the introduction of antipsychotic drugs, the modern colonies (asylums) have shrunk.

Corporate medicine's treatment for the schizophrenias demands that they are treated with the most current drugs. Many of these expensive new drugs are no better than the original antipsychotics that came into use in the 1950s; some even have increased side effects, such as metabolic syndrome and diabetes. One of the original antipsychotics, perphenazine, appears to be as effective and free of side effects as the modern drug olanzapine, but it costs far less.[16] While it might be expected that this would be welcome news, increasing medical cost effectiveness, psychiatrists are unimpressed with this study.

The importance of psychiatric drugs and therapies is that they lead the way for some of the gross abuses of power in modern medicine. Governments have a tendency to view psychiatry as a branch of policing and social control. Worldwide, there are numerous cases of dissident views being considered symptoms of mental illness. With diseases that are ill-defined, except for changes in behavior, it is easy for unwanted behavior to be considered aberrant, or even a sign of illness.

Psychiatric patients are often vulnerable and unable to defend their personal needs and boundaries. However, many other patients also face this challenge and can be victims of institutional abuse. A recent example is the use of antipsychotic medication in demented elderly patients. Elderly patients who suffer from Alzheimer's disease or similar dementia often display aberrant behavior. Some elderly patients, who are clear minded, may also be unwilling to accept the authority of the hospital and continue with unwanted behavior. There is thus pressure on hospital and other staff to tranquilize such patients and render them more malleable.

Some readers may think we are overstating the facts. Doctors, nurses and other health professionals work in hospitals for the benefit of the patients, and they consider their career a vocation. Surely, suggesting that they would give major tranquilizers to patients, risking serious side effects, merely to render them more manageable, is outlandish?

Unfortunately, this is not so. As we are writing this book, the abuse of antipsychotics to control the elderly has, at last, been picked up by the media.[17] The U.K. government initiated a review by Professor Sube Banerjee, of King's College, London. Dr. Banergee accepts that, for some patients, antipsychotic drugs would be necessary in the short term. In his view, they might be used for up to three months, when the patient is a danger to themselves or to others. Even this is a difficult moral question. For example, motorcycle racing could be considered dangerous or an exciting sport. If we take the former view, are we entitled to drug all would-be racers?

The U.K. National Health Service has been administering antipsychotics to 180,000 patients each year. Of these, only about 36,000 patients received any benefit. As a result of the drugs, there were 1,800 deaths and uncounted injuries from falls or through struggling following a stroke. In other words, a patient being given these drugs would have a 1 in 100 chance of dying (1,800/180,000) and a much greater risk of serious injury or side effects. So, for 20 people who needed the drug for some reason and benefited, one patient would be killed (1,800 compared with 36,000). Neil Hunt of the Alzheimer's Society said, "This goes beyond quality of care. It is a fundamental rights issue."

The abuse of major tranquilizers to chemically control the elderly is only one aspect of a failing system. A widespread issue is that care homes for the elderly are requiring feeding tubes to be surgically fitted, before a person can become a resident.[18] This is particularly the case with demented patients. The name "care homes" suggests a place of refuge, where a patient can expect to be properly fed. However, they appear to consider normal feeding a drain on resources. Perhaps the staff are simply too lazy to feed the patients? If technology can replace nursing, it may save time and effort, at the expense of depriving the unfortunate "inmates" of their last remaining pleasure.

Psychiatric patients admitted to mental hospitals in 1950 potentially faced a life sentence, with no time off for good behavior. In the past ten to twenty years, modern psychiatry adopted the corporate medicine point of view that, once a patient is on antipsychotic drugs, they should take them for life. One psychiatrist who recently advised a patient that he might be able to come off the drug was threatened with loss of his medical license. Fortunately, there is an increasing challenge to this viewpoint and the media is reporting the change.[19] Dr. William Carpenter, director of the University of Maryland's Psychiatric Research Center and editor of the journal *Schizophrenia Bulletin,* said, "My personal view is that the pendulum has swung too far and there's this knee jerk reaction out there that any period off medication, even for research, is on the face of it unethical."

Published clinical trials do not support the idea that patients on these drugs show greater healing. The lifetime medication creates huge numbers of dependent, chronic schizophrenic patients. Moreover, their chance of recovering decreases the longer that they stay on the drugs.

DIAGNOSING PSYCHOSIS

Early in Dr. Hoffer's long career as a psychiatrist he became aware of the need to diagnose schizophrenia accurately and reasonably quickly. In 1955, research psychologists had spent at least $50,000 to examine the clinical literature and concluded that there was no accurate test for this disease. They also decided that this was because psychiatrists would not agree on a definition and stick to it. The clinical expression of the disease was so variable that it was extremely difficult to sort it out from other conditions. This has been true of medicine in general. Syphilis had similarly varied symptoms and, until biological tests were developed, there was a similar degree of uncertainty in diagnosis.

The problems of diagnosing schizophrenia have not changed over the past fifty years. We still do not have any definitive test for the disease. The Minnesota Multiphasic Personality Inventory (MMPI) is a widely used psychological test used for diagnosis. The current test involves 567 questions. Clinically, it is of little value to the psychiatrist, even though it is used widely by psychologists. The accepted definition of schizophrenia and related disorders are specified in the American Psychiatric Association's *Diagnostic and Statistical Manual of Mental Disorders* (DSM, version DSM-IV-TR) and the World Health Organization's *International Statistical Classification of Diseases and Related Health Problems* (ICD-10). These definitions are not easily related to the results of the MMPI test.

Human beings are complicated individuals; while there may be specific characteristics of a disease such as schizophrenia they are unlikely to be captured and measured using a simple test. However, psychiatry needs objective methods to allow clinicians to agree on a diagnosis. The current diagnosis depends on the surface appearance of people: what people say and do are the measures used. All medical tests are uncertain and we suggest people do not take an assessment unless they have some signs of illness. As we have seen from the Rosenhan experiment, it is easy to be misdiagnosed and difficult to be reclassified as normal unless you admit to being insane. The paradoxical catch-22, from Joseph Heller's novel of the same name, applies. The Nobel Prize–winning physicist Richard Feynman was famous for his amusing stories in addition to his scientific accomplishments. However, he was classified as mentally unfit for the military after being assessed by a psychiatrist. Clearly sane and with an outstanding grasp of reality, Dr. Feynman had simply answered all the questions such as "Do you talk to yourself?" accurately and reasonably. Dr. Feynman's comment to the psychiatrist was telling: "And this is medicine?"[20]

The practice and science of psychiatry has been subjective and controversial. The DSM, often called "the psychiatrist's bible," is currently being updated, amid controversy. The diagnosis of mental illness is not scientific—it does not rest on direct measurement but relies on an interpretation of behavior. The new DSM-V will extend the definition of mental illness, bringing more people within the diagnostic criteria. Two psychiatrists, Drs. Robert Spitzer and Allen Frances, have strongly objected to the DSM update.[21] Dr. Frances was head of the panel that produced the previous version and he described the new version as a secretive process combining "the most unhappy combination of soaring ambition and weak methodology" with exaggerated claims.[22] We reproduce Frances's reservations here to clarify the problems.

- No scientific basis for the ambition to achieve a paradigm shift in the DSM.

- The absence of clear methodological guidelines and evidence for the changes.

- A lack of openness to wide scrutiny and useful criticism.

- An inability to spot the obvious dangers in most of their current proposals.

- The failure to set and meet timelines, and a likelihood of unconsidered last-minute decisions.

We encountered Dr. Spitzer earlier in this book, when he objected to

Rosenhan's research on getting healthy people admitted to mental hospitals. Here, he is again critical of the DSM committee, saying, "The main problem is that we don't know what they're doing."

A specific concern is that the DSM-V could include new categories of disease. Milder forms of aberrant behavior may be classified as illnesses such as schizophrenia, depression, or dementia. We all have minor personality deviations from the average. For example, a person with a tendency toward autism may be labeled as having Asperger's syndrome. However, in some groups, such as physicists or computer scientists, this trait is relatively common and useful. As the number of psychiatric conditions is expanded, it may be that people classified as normal or healthy become rare.[23] If this process continues, being normally sane could become a future illness and require medication. Dr. Frances suggests, "The result would be a wholesale . . . medicalization of normality that will lead to a deluge of unneeded medication." So, powerful antipsychotic drugs may be given before a person has experienced a psychotic episode if doctors predict they could be at risk of having one. This is clearly open to widespread abuse. It is not clear if such medication would be compulsory, as is common in cases of psychosis.

In his book *Indications of Insanity,* John Conolly (1794–1866) provided an alternative way of defining insanity.[24] Conolly's clear and elegant explanation is a useful working definition: insanity is a disease of perception, combined with an inability to tell whether these perceptual changes are real or not. Dr. Hoffer used this definition clinically and found it most valuable. Unfortunately, American psychiatry developed from an alternative definition of insanity described by Dr. Eugen Bleuler (1857–1939). His definition depended upon the presence or absence of thought disorder, with little emphasis given to perceptual changes. This remains a basis for diagnosis. It is difficult to define accurately when thought disorder is present. Moreover, we are in an age of multifactorial explanations in medicine, which reflects increasing uncertainty in our understanding.

Dr. Hoffer and Dr. Humphry Osmond created a simple test for assisting in the diagnosis of the schizophrenias, based upon the perceptual theory of schizophrenia: the Hoffer-Osmond Diagnostic (HOD) test.[25] The test consists of 145 cards, each containing a question to which the patient replies by placing the cards in a true or false category. The true questions are scored. Schizophrenics score high, usually over 50, while other persons

The HOD Diagnostic Test

The Hoffer-Osmond Diagnostic (HOD) test is a diagnostic tool of wide utility, developed initially in relation to schizophrenics. It is based on the idea that schizophrenia is an organic disease: that the intensity of the psychotic or neurotic manifestations are revealed by the degree that the senses (sight, hearing, taste, smell, etc.) are affected. Using responses from normal individuals as a baseline, a questionnaire (the HOD test) was created to reveal the kind and level of perceptual distortions experienced by patients. It consists of a series of cards with statements relevant to the perceptions, which the patient answers as "true" or "false." Here are a few statements from the HOD test:

- When I look at people they seem strange
- My thinking gets all mixed up when I have to act quickly
- Pictures appear to be alive and to breathe
- I can read other people's minds
- People's faces seem to change in size as I watch them
- I often hear or have heard voices talking about or to me
- People watch me all the time
- I often hear my thoughts inside my head
- I now become easily confused
- People's eyes seem very piercing and frightening
- Sometimes I feel very unreal
- I have to be on my guard with friends
- There is some plot against me
- At times my mind goes blank
- At times some other people can read my mind
- Some foods which never tasted funny before do so now
- I find that past, present, and future seem all muddled up

HOD testing consumes little time and can be accurately scored by almost anyone. A normal score was calculated to be under 40, but it was found that seriously ill schizophrenics could have scores ranging from 75 to as much as 150! Plus, the severity of the illness in its various mental and emotional manifestations could be readily diagnosed.

Dr. Hoffer's patients were routinely given the HOD test before being placed on niacin (vitamin B_3) therapy and other supportive medications. Two to three months later, when the patient again answered the identical questionnaire, his or her score had often made a noticeable drop toward normal. If niacin is withdrawn from treatment, after a similar period the HOD score often returns to the higher figure, and the patient appeared to be as sick as ever.

The HOD testing kit, along with full directions, can be obtained from: Behavior Science Press, 3710 Resource Drive, Tuscaloosa, AL 35401. Telephone: 800-826-7223, 205-758-2823, or 205-247-3134.

score low, usually under 30. The magnitude of the score indicates the likelihood one has schizophrenia.

There is also a skin test for schizophrenia developed by Dr. David Horrobin. Inspired by the work on niacin and schizophrenia, Dr. Horrobin realized that the skin flush caused by niacin might be an indicator of disease. Healthy people flush when given a large dose of niacin, but schizophrenic patients require a much higher dose to induce a flush. In the test, an adhesive strip containing four different concentrations of niacin is placed on the skin and left there for five minutes. The strip is then removed. Normally, the niacin in the patch will cause some reddening; a mild flush or dilatation at the point of contact. However, people with schizophrenia are more resistant to the effect.

This is a useful test, considering the difficulty in obtaining a diagnosis of schizophrenia and the absence of other physiological measures. There are some limitations, such as if a healthy person takes aspirin or a similar anti-inflammatory, the response may be absent as in a schizophrenic. The absence of a flush does not imply that a person is mentally ill. They may, for example, have a minor vitamin B_3 deficiency. However, the niacin patch is a straightforward physiological test. In a 1998 study of thirty-eight schizophrenics, the test gave a response in 83 percent of schizophrenics and only 23 percent of controls.[26] In a 2006 study, sixteen schizophrenics could be separated from seventeen depressed patients and sixteen controls based on skin flushing.[27] There have been several other studies showing the test can be effective.[28] The caveat is that the test is more predictive if there are pre-existing reasons for thinking a person is sick, such as a high score on a HOD test or strange behavior.

Psychiatry is currently based on subjective checklists and opinion. The niacin skin test is direct physiological indicator but typically is not used or even studied. This irrational behavior of psychiatrists could be seen as a refusal to change their current habits. The skin test would generally be seen as a breakthrough in providing a unique, physiological test for schizophrenia, but psychiatrists would need to directly address the problem with the biochemistry of niacin in schizophrenics.

NUTRITIONAL THERAPY FOR PSYCHOSIS

Caught early, psychosis responds well to treatment. The longer the person has been sick and the greater the number of psychotic episodes, the slower is the recovery. Chronic schizophrenic patients respond slowly to nutritional treatment—it may take up to ten years before the maximum benefit is seen. From a recent survey of about 500 chronic patients under Dr. Hoffer's care, he concluded that the major recovery occurred about five to seven years after treatment was initiated.[29] If nutritional supplementation is discontinued too soon, the optimum therapeutic effect will not be seen.

One of the problems with psychiatric hospitals is that they stop the nutritional therapy when a patient is admitted. It is as if the psychiatrists are demanding authority over all aspects of the patient's care. On the rare occasions when Dr. Hoffer's patients were admitted, the hospital doctors promptly stopped his nutritional program, prescribed medication, and took away the patient's vitamins. A few determined patients had their families smuggle the vitamins into the hospital or surreptitiously took the supplements on their own. If the patient were found out, the hospital might assume this behavior is a symptom, rather than a rational response. Forbidding the use of supplements interrupts treatment and retards recovery. Patients chose to return to Dr. Hoffer when they were discharged and began their nutritional therapy again.

Chronic psychiatric patients must be treated patiently and continuously, with adequate support. A combination of short-term medication and long-term nutrient therapy combines the advantages of the rapid effect of drugs and the slow, curative effect of the nutrients. This permits a gradual reduction of medication, until the dose is so low the drug no longer creates its tranquilizer psychosis. Schizophrenia in children may take the form of a learning disorder, so normally intelligent persons appear retarded. Lifting the psychosis by means of orthomolecular therapy will remove the apparent learning difficulty.

The orthomolecular therapy for psychosis consists of taking sufficient niacin, vitamin C, and perhaps fish oils. Schizophrenics need greater intakes of niacin than normal people. Sufficient niacin and vitamin C, perhaps 2–3 grams of each spread throughout the day, will gradually return most schizophrenics to normality.

Dr. Hoffer's criteria for recovery are simple:

• There must be no symptoms and signs.

• The patient must be getting on well with family.

One of a Kind

Dr. David Horrobin (1939–2003) was one of the most original scientific minds in nutrition and physiology. At Balliol College, Oxford, he obtained a science degree with First Class Honors; to this, he added a medical degree and a doctorate in neuroscience.

Medical pioneers are not happy with the standard methods of treatment taught in medical school. They have the initiative to try to improve the available treatments with true scientific medicine. Fortunately for schizophrenic patients, Dr. Horrobin became dissatisfied with the results of modern psychiatry. Dr. Hoffer first heard him as a young scientist at a meeting of the Canadian Schizophrenia Foundation in Montreal. Dr. Hoffer had described how schizophrenics given niacin typically did not flush, and Dr. Horrobin immediately realized the implications and asked a question from the floor. It is notable that no one else had ever referred to that observation. David Horrobin realized that a lack of the niacin flush might be a physiological indicator of psychosis.

A few years later, Dr. Horrobin became particularly interested in the role of the essential fatty acids (EFAs) found in fish oil. He was a fellow of Magdalen College, where he taught medicine alongside Dr. Hugh Sinclair, one of

- The patient must be getting on well with the community.

- The patient must be employed, i.e., paying income taxes.

The nutritional therapy is effective and patients recover, whereas corporate psychiatry provides remarkably little help to patients beyond tranquilizing them. One of the advantages of the orthomolecular approach is that patients are more compliant, since they do not suffer major drug side effects. When drugs are needed, the dose is small and side effects are minimized or avoided.

Niacin: An Antipsychotic Nutrient

Jim had been totally unmanageable. At twenty-one, he'd already been kicked out of the state hospital for being too violent. They sent him home to his parents, whom he threatened on a daily basis, while punching holes

---

the pioneers in the field of EFAs. Dr. Horrobin became increasingly fascinated in lipid biochemistry and its role in human disease. From his travels in East Africa and work in Kenya, he developed new ideas about fatty acids, schizophrenia, and its role in evolution. He described these ideas in his book *The Madness of Adam and Eve*. His interest and drive persuaded universities to test his ideas that these fatty acids could help in treatment. Unlike many lesser scientists, Dr. Horrobin realized that more than one biochemical defect was involved in psychosis. He thought that there would be a simple solution to schizophrenia and that patients could be quickly returned to normal. His scientific interests were wide-ranging, leading him to be frustrated by the slow pace of research and by so-called evidence-based medicine. He was critical of multimillion-dollar treatment trials, pointing out that these were needed only when the drug being tested hardly worked at all. Dr. Horrobin founded two medical journals which expanded on this scientific philosophy: *Medical Hypotheses* and *Prostaglandins, Leukotrienes and Essential Fatty Acids*.

As is common with exceptional scientists Dr. Horrobin made many professional friends and some enemies. On his death, the *British Medical Journal* published an unpleasant and critical obituary of him. The journal immediately received many letters of protest from his former colleagues and supporters all over the world. We need more scientists like David Horrobin.

in the livingroom walls. Jim slept one hour per night and roamed the streets for the other seven. His face was scaly and severely broken out with acne. His dietary and digestive habits were appalling.

Corporate medicine had failed Jim and his parents. Dr. Saul told them about Dr. Hoffer's approach: take very large quantities of niacin, starting at 3,000 milligrams a day, plus an equal or larger amount of vitamin C. Advanced niacin deficiency, or pellagra, causes psychosis, as well as the skin and gastrointestinal problems that Jim was experiencing. He needed more niacin than an average person. In large doses, niacin has a profound calming and sedating effect. Niacin is powerful, but it is not a drug, it is a nutrient. Its safety margin is large—Dr. Hoffer has, on occasion, prescribed 20,000 mg or more a day.

About two weeks later, Jim's father called. "Let me tell you what happened," he began. "You know Jim only sleeps maybe an hour a night? Well, the first night on the niacin, he slept eighteen hours. He's been sleeping about seven hours a night since."

"That's terrific," said Dr. Saul.

"That's not all," he said. "Last Friday morning, for the first time in I don't know how many years, Jim came down for breakfast. He walked into the dining room and said 'Good morning, Dad.'"

Even on the phone, Dr. Saul could hear the tears in the man's voice. It was wonderful news.

Niacin toxicity is rare. Doctors frequently give patients 2,000–5,000 mg of niacin to lower serum cholesterol. Dr. Hoffer estimated that over about 200,000 mg per day could be fatal. These levels are far higher than people supplementing with niacin are likely to try.

Most healthy people will not exceed an intake of 1,000 mg without having a severe flush. A large dose of niacin, especially if taken on an empty stomach, will cause a flush: the skin reddens and this blushing gradually spreads over the whole body. The red skin can be accompanied by a pleasant tingling sensation or a strong feeling of burning. Either way, the reaction is harmless. The feeling of burning usually occurs in those who have a flush without being prepared for the reaction. Most people adapt to the flush quite quickly after a few attempts, and some even come to enjoy it.

Niacin is safe when compared with drugs. Even widely available over-the-counter drugs are far more dangerous, causing many deaths every year.

In comparison, there is not even one death from niacin each year. The flush can lower body temperature, especially on a cold day. Such symptoms vary with dose and the body's need. Slowing down the absorption by taking niacin after a meal may prevent the flushing and associated side effects. The upper limit is the amount that causes nausea and the dose should be lowered if this occurs.

People with a history of heavy alcohol use, liver disorders, diabetes, or pregnancy need to have their physician monitor their use of high-dose niacin. Monitoring long-term use of niacin is a good idea for anyone on high intakes. A doctor can check your liver function with a simple blood test. Note that niacin therapy increases liver function tests, but this elevation indicates that the liver is more metabolically active; it does not necessarily indicate an underlying liver pathology. Many compounds elevate liver enzymes, including common drugs such as statins, paracetamol (acetaminophen or Tylenol), and ibuprofen (Advil). Unless the increase with niacin is substantial, say threefold higher, it may not be clinically important. Negative side effects are easily dealt with by physicians who are familiar with niacin. Some of the side effects may be minimized with vitamin C, as they may be a result of low antioxidant status.

Positive side effects of niacin are not often covered by corporate medicine. Niacin will increase general health, improve healing, and prolong a high quality of life. In sharp contrast, few drugs have positive side effects. Lack of niacin is a major public health problem. The U.S. Recommended Dietary Allowance (RDA) for niacin is only about 20 mg. About half of all Americans will not get even that much from their diets.[30] However, the bodily need for niacin varies with activity, body size, and illness.

Of course, not every psychiatric patient wants or is willing to take niacin and vitamin C. Sometimes, they will take it for unlikely reasons; for example, Dr. Hoffer once convinced a psychiatric patient with painful earwax that a niacin flush would help melt the wax and keep his ears clean. This was an unusual way of convincing the patient, but it worked: the patient's earwax softened and, as a side effect, he stopped being psychotic.

One female patient refused to take her niacin and vitamin C, and she gradually became more psychotic. She would not visit Dr. Hoffer and refused any medical treatment. In an increasing rage with her mother's persistent pleas that she needed help, the daughter decided to commit suicide. She told the mother she had had enough and would show her and that doctor. She grabbed the bottle of niacin tablets and attempted to overdose, swallowing and chewing the tablets, and pushing the mother away. The mother relaxed, made herself a cup of coffee, and waited. The daughter had a massive niacin flush and gradually calmed down. Of course, the niacin did not kill or harm her—it just helped her recover her sanity. The daughter apologized and went back on her nutrient therapy.

Success Story: Elizabeth

Often, discussion of psychiatric problems can be a little impersonal. However, each psychosis can destroy a person or even a whole family. Here, we describe the case of Elizabeth, one of Dr. Hoffer's patients.

Elizabeth came to see Dr. Hoffer in December 1995. Her family practitioner wrote in his referral letter, "She is twenty-eight years old with a long history of psychiatric illness, with varied diagnosis, including anorexia nervosa, borderline personality disorder, multiple personality disorder, and these are associated with suicide attempts and multiple hospitalizations." Elizabeth had also been diagnosed with depression.

About mid-1992, she began to suffer severe headaches. These migraines occurred two to three times per month, were unrelated to her periods, and were often preceded by nausea and vomiting. She had been given the usual variety of headache medication, without any response, including Fiorinal, Demerol, Gravol, Tylenol, and Imitrex by injection. Her general practitioner had reported to the neurologist that she was working as a nurse's aid; Elizabeth was a good worker and hated missing work.

Elizabeth had been a member of an eating disorder support group. When she was sixteen, she would starve herself for up to six weeks. Then, after having gained some weight, she would resume her fasting. She had also used laxatives as an aid to weight loss. Later, she began to use medication such as Ionamin to control her appetite. Elizabeth would binge and vomit three or four times per week; sometimes, she would eat and vomit twice each day. This behavior has the immediate side effect of preventing the absorption of brain-protective nutrients such as vitamins B and C. She had been an excellent student and a good athlete, happy with school and with her family.

Early in 1993, a consultant reported that Elizabeth had an eating disorder that was not responding to treatment. For over three weeks, she had fasted and drank little fluids. She felt faint, had palpitations, and was tired.

She was admitted to the hospital a second time, with severe depression, auditory hallucinations, and suicidal ideas. On this admission, Elizabeth admitted she had been a victim of child sexual abuse, by her stepfather. She continued to hear voices, a clear symptom of psychosis, but the psychiatrist in charge interpreted these as a projection of her own thoughts. He began to indulge in psychoanalytic speculations about the causes of Elizabeth's voices, which he denied were hallucinations. Such speculation on the part of the doctor is irrational. Nutrient deficiency was clearly present and can result in psychosis and depression.

For the first time, the term *personality disorder* began to appear in her record. A personality disorder is a chronic personality style that is unresponsive to medication. The most well-known form of personality disorder is the psychopath. The suggestion of a personality disorder was in striking contrast to the opinion of her general practitioner, who had seen Elizabeth as basically a normal, achieving person. She was diagnosed with depression and placed on antidepressants.

About six months before seeing Dr. Hoffer, Elizabeth was assessed by psychologists. She reported hearing derogatory voices inside her head, which had become louder in the past few years. She also heard voices from outside, calling her. She hallucinated faces in several different and visually complex scenes and places, such as in flowers, food, and in a window. Furthermore, she reported having been in four car accidents due to blackouts when driving. It was suggested that she suffered from dissociative reactions, such as daydreaming and amnesia, but no specific diagnosis was made.

During Elizabeth's first interview with Dr. Hoffer, she complained she had been depressed and agitated for four years. She was less depressed while on Prozac but was still having problems with her eating disorder. A mental state examination confirmed a variety of perceptual symptoms, including hearing voices of several men and seeing visions, and there was also a change in taste perception. Importantly, she could not tell the difference between the hallucinations and real phenomena. She was also very paranoid and suspicious of her family and friends.

Dr. Hoffer disregarded the previous diagnoses, which ignored her major symptoms, and diagnosed her as schizophrenic. He used the Hoffer-Osmond Diagnostic (HOD) test for assisting in the diagnosis of the schizophrenia.[31] Elizabeth scored 152 on the HOD test, suggesting severe psychosis. Dr. Hoffer assessed the odds Elizabeth was schizophrenic at over 90 percent.

He started her on niacin (500 mg) and vitamin C (1,000 mg), three times a day. To this were added daily doses of vitamin B_6 (pyridoxine) (250 mg) and zinc citrate (50 mg). Elizabeth was asked to go on an ortho-molecular diet of unprocessed, whole foods, along with the restriction of dairy products, little sugar, and no junk food as part of her therapy.[32]

Three months later, Elizabeth was free of voices. A month after that, Dr. Hoffer heard from the referring physician, expressing his pleasure at seeing how well she was. He added, "She is almost unrecognizably improved." By June of the following year, both Elizabeth and Dr. Hoffer agreed that she had greatly improved. She stated that she felt normal for the first time in five years. In July, she visited her mother with her three children and enjoyed the visit. When she had been depressed and paranoid, her psychiatrist had stated that she had a poor relationship with her parents. This was no longer the case. Her HOD scores were now normal. Elizabeth remained on niacin (4,500 mg each day), Prozac (20 mg a day), and the rest of the vitamin regimen.

After Elizabeth was properly diagnosed and given the correct nutritional treatment, she was almost normal in a few months. She returned from the state of a person declared inadequate, suffering an untreatable personality disorder, severe depression, and migraine headaches, to the normal individual she had been before her illness. Finally, she was now a person, not a patient.

PART TWO

. . . .

Antidote— Patient Power

CHAPTER 6

The Hospital Game

"Never ask a barber if you need a haircut."
—Warren Buffet

Staying healthy involves making a series of decisions. Decision science explains how people can make rational decisions. One aspect of decision science, game theory, suggests we should take a paranoid approach to the kind of one-off decisions necessary in hospitals. This means you should always act to maximize your own benefit and, more importantly, to minimize your biggest risk of harm. A rational patient will ruthlessly demand the treatments that minimize their risk of suffering serious injury. In short, a patient must be risk averse. Clearly, the same applies to doctors, who should always avoid taking risks with patients.

The discipline and applications of game theory were highly influenced by the mathematician John Nash, made famous by the book and film *A Beautiful Mind*. However, Nash was a paranoid schizophrenic and his view of the world was odd. He and other early game theorists believed that every one was selfish, scheming, and acting in their own personal interest. Nash's paranoia was particularly useful in the game theory mindset. According to game theory, we should all act rather like paranoid sociopaths. This might be a rather frightening prospect if it ever came to pass. Fortunately, we live in a world mostly populated by normal, rational, and caring human beings. As a theoretical construct, however, game theory is a powerful technique and is used effectively in many contexts, such as the military, politics, big business, and medical management.

Patients can apply game theory to doctors, nurses, hospitals, and corporate medicine. Professionals, such as lawyers and accountants, and organizations, such as banks, try to behave rationally. Since that is the case, their behavior can be modeled rather accurately by considering them to be selfish and mean. We can assume their main concern is for their own benefit and they are far less concerned about the harm they might do to others. The recent problems with the financial system might be considered a vindication of this view—investment bankers maximized their personal gain at enormous cost to the economy and taxpayers.

CORPORATE MEDICINE'S GAME

It is rational for patients to be paranoid about corporate medicine and hospitals. The old joke that "just because you are paranoid doesn't mean they aren't out to get you" applies. Similarly, in the current system, hospitals and doctors often feel paranoid about litigious patients and their lawyers. We don't need to extend this kind of thinking to our everyday lives but, in the hospital, our lives are at risk. If we were more paranoid by nature, we could invent a scenario in which the leaders of major drug companies get together in expensive resorts to develop the criteria for selling drugs with maximum profit. Each chief executive officer (CEO) has an obligation to maximize their company's profits; their official role is to generate profit for shareholders. However, game theory suggests the chief executives' actual aim will be maximizing their own personal benefit. Therefore, companies harness individual aims by giving share options to personnel, so that what is good for the company is good for the executive. Of course, if the CEOs did get together to maximize profits, this would be an illegal cartel, a price-fixing conspiracy. In practice, they do not need to conspire in this way. They just need to have a feel for the market—groupthink and conformity will do the rest.

Corporate medicine has some straightforward requirements for their products. These are rational and can be predicted using game theory. Our CEOs in their exclusive hideaway might suggest an ideal drug should have the following characteristics:

• It would give some therapeutic benefit—perhaps not too much, but enough that the patient wants to keep taking the drug.

• It must not cure the patient entirely, as they would then have no further need for the drug, which would hurt profits.

- The drug should be addictive or be widely used for a chronic condition, leading to more sales.

- If use is not long term, the drug should be capable of attracting a high value (e.g., expensive anti-cancer drugs).

- Side effects must not be apparent in controlled trials (with the exception of anti-cancer drugs).

Many recently developed drugs (not to mention illegal recreational substances) meet these criteria; a classic example would be statins. Is this pure chance? A conspiracy? Or does this result emerge naturally from a system devised to make money from sick people? We think the latter is the case. Corporate medicine is constructed as a branch of commerce and, as such, the results will inevitably work against patients' best interests.

ROLE-PLAYING AS DOCTORS AND PATIENTS

Throughout this book, we are critical of corporate medicine and hospitals in particular. This does not extend to individual physicians. Many physicians working in the system are ethical and care about their patients; they would not knowingly harm a patient. It is not the individual doctors that are the issue but the organization of medicine.

Medicine and other professions are distinguished by monopolization of specialist knowledge along with considerable freedom from accountability.[1] It used to be the case that doctors typically had an automatic authority over patients. However, patients are becoming more educated and, with the advent of the Internet, have access to similar information to that of the specialist. Patients are expecting a higher standard of care and more respect from their doctors. A medical consultation is starting to resemble a negotiation.

Negotiation is a process by which people with conflicting interests determine how they are going to allocate resources or work together in the future.[2] *Every interaction between a patient and a doctor is a negotiation.* As a patient, your interests may include receiving treatment, health care, and reassurance. The physician's concerns may include taking account of other patients, adhering to standard medical practice, and getting paid. As in any negotiation, there are rules you can apply to help you achieve the optimal outcome.

The interaction between doctor and patient can be considered according to the rules of game theory. This allows us to break down the two roles and consider their respective goals. The use of the word *game* does not imply that we are trying to trivialize the interaction. Game theory relates to decision making in a competitive situation and aims to find the "best" or optimal course of action.[3] Researchers originally applied the theory to games such as poker, chess, and bridge. Its later development was intimately associated with military strategy and the Cold War. More recently, applications in the behavioral sciences have been analyzed, particularly in economics.

In this chapter, we are concerned with the "hospital game," during which a patient attempts to negotiate the best outcome for their health and well-being with health professionals. The hospital game generally involves role playing: one person acts as patient and another takes the role of physician. Conventional strategies are expected of these roles, which may help the hospital more than the patient.

The doctor role includes acting as gatekeeper to health-care resources. As such, doctors behave in ways that would be utterly inappropriate in other settings: asking intimate questions of people they hardly know or requiring patients to remove clothes and submit to physical examinations. Likewise, if the patient wants access to health care, they may feel obliged to answer questions and allow intrusions that, in a different context, might be seen as interrogation or even torture. Under these circumstances, it helps to remember that both you (the patient) and the medical staff are people.

A patient often has a specific goal: perhaps he is suffering from a particular symptom and his hopes include being reassured that it is not serious, receiving treatment, and recovering. If the patient pays for medical services directly, he may also want to know that he can afford them. He may perform a simple cost-benefit analysis; perhaps he estimates that removal of an annoying wart is worth, say, $50. By contrast, if he has terminal cancer, he may be willing to spend his whole life savings, on top of any medical insurance. The massive personal cost of some conditions means that patients are vulnerable and could be exploited by unscrupulous people or quacks offering ineffective therapies.

In an ideal world, the physician's interests would coincide exactly with those of the patient. In reality, the physician has to balance a complicated set of constraints, in addition to his own personal goals, any of which may conflict with the wishes of the patient. Legally, for example, physicians are limited as to which medicines they can prescribe and when they can provide them. Additionally, their actions are restricted by a set of expectations from their profession, which specify what is considered as "best practice." Any deviation from standard practice might not break the

Taking Back Control

The hospital is organized to place patients in a position of relative weakness. Hospitals do not rely on the disparity in resources, information, and expertise, but have other mechanisms of social control. The waiting for the doctor to "see you now," the white coats and even the use of the labels "doctor" and "nurse" are mechanisms of control and roles that are played.

One patient in an English hospital described how they objected to providing their first, or Christian, name to a nurse. They indicated that they did not appreciate people in big organizations being disrespectful. The response was telling. The nurse replied, "We are taught in training always to ask to use a patient's first name, because that puts us in charge."[4]

Make the staff call you by your formal name, such as Mrs. Smith. This makes it clear that you have some relevant status as an intelligent adult and are not simply a patient. If they wish to be called by their title, they should have reciprocal respect. Your social position is of some concern to staff in a hospital and is likely to make a difference to the care you receive.

Unnecessary operations, which can be highly lucrative, are increasing. By 1992, over 17 percent of surgeries in the United States were based on unconfirmed diagnoses, and 2.4 million unnecessary operations were performed annually, with approximately 11,900 deaths, at a cost of $3.9 billion.[5] These patients would have done well to ensure that their surgery was really necessary. In cases where surgery is elective, such as breast enhancement or a nose job, the patient needs to make sure that they have balanced the costs and benefits carefully. In particular, it is important to get an estimate of the risk of major negative outcomes, so the patient can do a simple worst-case analysis.

In the hospital game, patients should adopt a paranoid attitude—do not assume that everything is as it appears.

law but could exceed the terms of their medical license, their medical insurance, or open them up to the risk of being sued. Such behavior could also lead to professional censure, which is a powerful constraint. Private medical practitioners need to cover their costs, including overhead, staff, and insurance. So, a doctor may view her patients as customers as well as patients.

SELF-SERVING ADVICE

Health professionals frequently release health care advice, which is claimed to be for the benefit of patients. An example is to use elastic stockings on long airplane flights to prevent deep vein thrombosis (DVT). Thrombosis can occur when blood flow is reduced, a blood vessel wall is damaged, or spontaneously in some people, who have an abnormal tendency for blood clotting. DVT can be life-threatening, especially in the legs: about 3 in 100 people with clots in their lower limbs will die. The risk of an adult having a DVT increases by 12 percent when one long flight is taken each year.[6] In the two weeks after the flight, the risk is about four times higher. However, the risk of death from a DVT on a flight is small compared with accidents at work or motor vehicle fatalities.

Since sitting motionless for long periods can increase risk, the standard medical advice to wear elastic socks and, especially, to move about on long flights is sensible. Unfortunately, the advice is also self-serving and the widespread emphasis on flying distracts attention from a greater cause of DVT. In a hospital bed, you are often immobile for far longer than a long flight and the risks of DVT are correspondingly greater.

Here, we use the risk of DVT in the hospital as a practical example of how negotiation may save your life. While a long trip on an airplane increases risk of DVT slightly, hospital patients are at much greater risk. The increased risk for major venous blood clots in the hospital is large for surgery (twenty-two times higher than normal), trauma (thirteen times higher), and hospital or nursing home confinement (eight times higher).[7] In this case, conventional medicine has given air travel a bad name, while hiding a higher risk that is directly attributable to themselves.

Lifeblood, a thrombosis charity in the U.K., suggests that harmful clotting affects about 1 in 1,000 people each year.[8] A similar risk is associated with pregnancy. Of those affected, one in ten will die if untreated. However, Lifeblood also states that, unless preventive measures are taken, one in three surgical patients may develop DVT. Lifeblood's figures for DVT in the hospital are as follows[9]:

- 17 in 100 chance if you are ill on a medical ward

- 50-50 chance if you are on the ward with a severe stroke

- Greater than 50-50 chance for an orthopedic operation on the hip

- Almost certain (nearly 100 percent chance) in a case of severe trauma

It is estimated that that one in ten hospital deaths are caused by abnormal venous clotting.[10] The number of people dying from hospital-induced DVT is five times greater than the number who die from hospital-acquired infections. These deaths could be avoided with clinical awareness, preventive medicine, and good nutrition. Hospitals are killing patients through lack of basic care.

The fact that you are asked to take precautions before flying in an airplane but not before entering the hospital is worrying. You need to protect yourself from this major cause of death—you cannot rely on the medical staff. Consider using both nutritional supplements and negotiation skills. If possible, before a hospital stay, make sure that you are not at high risk of inappropriate blood clotting. To do this, you can take supplements of vitamin C (3,000 mg) and fish oils (2,000 mg); also helpful are vitamin E, NAC (N-acetyl-cysteine), and possibly the herbs ginger and *Ginkgo biloba*. Take these nutrients in the weeks leading up to a hospital stay. Good nutrition may prevent the abnormal clotting and save your life. Unfortunately, the medical professionals who are negligent in preventing hospital deaths by DVT may often try to prevent your use of supplementation.

Before admission to a hospital, you might ask: "Will I be at risk of DVT during my stay and how do you propose preventing its occurrence?" and "What is the risk of DVT during my stay?" If you do not get an educated response to these questions, reconsider your choice of hospital. Typical suggestions include use of anti-embolism stockings or pneumatic compression boots, if you are likely to be bedridden for a prolonged period. Also, ask if the hospital has ultrasound facilities that will be used to check for DVTs. If you are unfortunate enough to suffer a DVT, it is reassuring to know that the hospital can diagnose it correctly. By asking such questions, you are informing the hospital staff that you are aware of the DVT issue and increasing the likelihood that the staff will be predisposed to prevention and diagnosis of the condition.

One approach the hospital may suggest is the use of blood thinners, drugs such as warfarin, to prevent blood clotting. However, such drugs can cause unnecessary bleeding, hemorrhage, and stroke. Artificial prevention of clotting with drugs also has associated risks. If the hospital suggests blood thinners, you should proceed with care. You might begin by asking: "Before using drugs, are you proposing to check my blood clotting to see if I am at high risk?" You need to be sure that you only use anti-embolism drugs if they will substantially reduce the risks to your health.

In addition to knowing that you are being administered such drugs because your blood is prone to clotting, you need to check how they are going to monitor your blood. Blood clotting is an incredibly complex mechanism, which facilitates wound healing while preventing internal clotting such as DVT. It is not possible to simply take a drug and modify blood clotting safely, without constant checking. Their proposal should include monitoring your blood frequently while you are in the hospital. A simple fish oil supplement can prevent the need for warfarin treatment. Get the doctor's opinion on trying fish oil and high doses of vitamin C and rechecking your clotting before you elect to use the drug.

Also, ask about the side effects of the blood-thinning drug and its interactions with other medications and food. Warfarin, for example, has a long list of interactions and restrictions. Finally, you need to ask how long they propose you will stay on blood-thinning medication. Consider their response carefully—the drug interactions will affect you for the time you are on the drug, and you will need to be monitored frequently and consistently over the period you are medicated. There are costs, both monetary and in restrictions on your lifestyle.

Healthy people who take appropriate nutritional supplements can expect to have normal blood clotting and a lower risk of hospital-induced death by DVT. They can thus avoid the risk both of DVT and the blood-thinning drugs. Take control of your health. Hospitals cause this problem, so don't look to them for a solution.

CONFLICTS OF INTEREST

With any professional who provides advice or services, there is likely to be a conflict of interest. In most decisions, there will be influences that may not act in the patient's best interests. For example, a doctor may recommend a diagnostic test that is not really necessary, and may even have an associated risk, because performing the test may reduce his or her risk of liability.

In the U.S., the use of "managed care," which claims to reduce the cost of providing health benefits while improving the quality of care, means the doctor's options may be restricted.[11] They may have a limited number and type of treatments and conditions under which they are provided. One drug may have less risk of side effects but may be much more expensive. The choice may come down to the cost.

Medicine involves complicated decision making, and the decision may have financial implications for the doctor. For example, telling a patient the results of a simple test over the telephone may prevent the costs of an office visit, which may be more advantageous for the patient than the doctor. However, some test results may be upsetting and require detailed explanation; if this happens, you may decide a face-to-face meeting was worth the cost.

THE BALANCE OF POWER

It is often assumed that physicians require authority in the doctor-patient relationship.[12] This sovereignty of medical doctors is a relatively new phenomenon. In the mid-1800s, medicine was a despised profession. However, the sick and their relatives are often emotional and vulnerable and may not be the most rational judges. In addition to their professional knowledge, doctors are often thought to have particular skill in decision making. While doctors exercise control over patients, other health-care workers, and the general public, they are not trained in decision science nor do they necessarily have great judgment. Patients need to think for themselves.

Trust is essential in the patient-doctor relationship, but this should not translate into giving doctors unwarranted power. We place similar trust in a bus driver or airline pilot to take us safely to our destination. Often, we might not be interested in the details of the route. However, taxi drivers can take long detours to hike up the fare. With doctors, "we must trust that our vulnerabilities will not be exploited for power, profit, prestige, or pleasure."[13] The more power given to the doctor, the greater is the patient's vulnerability. Patients must bear some of the responsibility for

For Your Own Good?

Imagine a fifty-five-year-old woman has cancer of the uterus and is given the option for potentially life-saving surgery. The surgery involves removing the ovaries and fallopian tubes, rendering her sterile. At first, she agrees to have the procedure, and then she changes her mind. The woman claims she has a fear of hospitals and particularly needles. The cancer is slow-growing, but without the surgery it will probably spread and kill her.

Should she be forced to have the surgery for her own good? By force, we mean should she be tricked into taking a drug to sedate her in her own home. Then, she would be transferred to the hospital and operated on. If necessary, after the operation she would be physically restrained and drugged to prevent her leaving the hospital before she has fully recovered. We expect most readers would consider this option unethical, authoritarian, and unjustified. It would clearly be assault against the poor woman.

Now, what if the woman had "learning difficulties." Does this mean that she should be forced to have the surgery? After all, if you arrive in an emergency room unconscious after an automobile accident, the medical team will make decisions on your behalf, including the decision to operate. Similar situations arise where doctors make decisions for drunk, psychotic, confused, or demented patients. So, do learning difficulties and a reported significant impairment in intellectual functioning mean that she can be treated in this way?

A judge in the United Kingdom has recently given doctors this option in a case.[14] The judge deemed that the woman was incapable of making a rational decision and such action was in her best interests.[15] The mandated surgery might cure the cancer, but then again it might not. The woman was accused of failing to attend hospital appointments, which implies that she was expected to have sufficient intellect to manage this action. Notably, her initial decision to have the operation was considered rational and acceptable, while changing her mind was not. Her ability to make the decision was questioned when she gave the "wrong" answer. Under the circumstances, the woman's phobia is well founded, since avoiding hospitals would be one way of maintaining her autonomy rather than being drugged and assaulted against her will. Her second specific phobia was against needles—intravenous needles would be inserted into this poor woman and held in place by bandages. We have known suicides to occur with far less stress.

Now, consider a patient with cancer wishing to try a treatment based on vitamin C. The doctors decide that the patient should have standard chemotherapy instead. Importantly, they might consider the patient to be irrational to choose vitamin C rather than chemotherapy. It might be concluded that a patient displaying such absurdity is incapable of making a rational decision. In this case, even if the patient had a doctoral degree in science it might not help, as the incapacity could be deemed to be madness rather than incapacity.

One woman posted the following eloquent response to the *Daily Telegraph* newspaper's website after reading this woman's story:

"I too have a phobia about hospitals and have refused further surgery. This is not because of mental impairment, but because of the incompetence, negligence, arrogance, and aggression that I have suffered from doctors and nurses in two London hospitals to date. . . . I went into hospital relatively healthy and thanks to their 'skills' am left disfigured and physically ill for life. To me, it makes perfect sense that I would not want such shysters anywhere near me again, yet the medics cannot understand the logic of it. The woman featured in this article will inevitably be made ill by the surgery and treatment for cancer. She could have legitimately decided that she would rather not undergo that. She emphatically should not have been forced to do so."[16]

When is it irrational to exercise your rational choice?

the incredibly high rate of adverse events in medicine. We need to demand higher standards and greater care.

Having authority over patients makes doctors feel important. It can also give them freedom to make a suboptimal decision with your life and health; they make the decision and you take the consequences. You have more control over your health and medical interventions than you might realize. To exercise this control, it is necessary to make sure you know as much as possible about your condition before discussing your options with the doctor.

Doctors and other medical professionals need your consent before they provide treatment. Consent may be assumed if you are unconscious or unable to respond. In special cases, such as children, or people suffering from psychosis or dementia, the problem of consent is more complicated. However, in general, you have ultimate control and can veto the proposed treatment, if you so decide. The doctor has a duty to act in your interests and to warn patients about the risks of treatment.

INTERVIEW YOUR DOCTOR

You want to find a rational doctor who puts your interests ahead of those of corporate medicine. Your goal is to find someone who values patient choice and true participation. Such a doctor might be a person who has the following characteristics:

- Is supportive of holistic or alternative forms of medicine

- Takes a patient-centered approach

- Communicates risks as well as advantages of treatment

- Respects the patient

- Involves the patient in decisions

- Describes the illness or problem in straightforward language

- Believes preventive medicine is more important than treatment

- Uses the fewest drugs possible

- Does not insist on medical screening without prior indications or symptoms

- Understands high-dose vitamin supplementation

- Will not force you or your children to have vaccinations if you choose not to

Selecting a doctor requires careful evaluation. For example, not all doctors who promote themselves as "holistic" or "alternative" will be as advertised; paying lip-service to a natural health philosophy is not the same as practicing it. Look for membership in appropriate professional bodies or capitalize on other people's experience with a particular doctor by asking around. People at a complementary health center may be familiar with many of these issues and be able to provide information on the attitude of local doctors.

You can screen any physician you are considering to trust with your health. If there is a charge for an initial consultation, then ask the office manager, nurse, or assistant for information. You need a positive response to your questions. Of course, you can terminate the discussion at any time if feedback is not consistent with your requirements. The screening process is a negotiation, and you have the final say.

You will have to decide on a list of characteristics that are important to you. However, taking the list above as an example, you might proceed as follows. If the response to your questions about preventive medicine is positive, then ask the doctor about her approach to health. Explain that you are looking for a doctor who will work in partnership with you, but agrees that, ultimately, you are in charge of your own health. You need to know if this personal control is compatible with the physician's philosophy of care.

You could tell the doctor that you take vitamin supplements and ask how she feels about that. An ideal response might be that she is fully supportive and considers it a wise form of medical insurance. An unacceptable response might be that you can get all the vitamins and minerals you need from five helpings of fruits and vegetables a day. We have also known doctors who denounce taking supplements as "quackery," saying that they do no good, probably do harm, and merely support unscrupulous purveyors of vitamins. However, when asked, not one of these critics has been able to provide suitable evidence.

The often-controversial issue of immunization provides useful insight in selecting your doctor. If you did not wish to have immunizations for yourself or your child, would the physician be willing to accept this viewpoint? The physician is likely to respond that immunization has helped relegate infectious diseases to the past. This degree of protection for the population depends upon a high proportion of people being immunized to prevent the spread of infectious diseases. However, game theory tells us that the rational patient acts for their own benefit, not misguided altruism. Moreover, there are scientists who do not agree with these generalized claims for vaccination. An alternative explanation is the decline in infectious disease arose from improvements in sanitation and nutrition.

Some people object to the mumps, measles, and rubella (MMR) combined vaccination, and there is no reason why these vaccinations cannot be given separately. The medical industries have persisted in putting mer-

Do I Really Need a Heart Bypass?

Many people with angina or related heart disease opt for bypass surgery. Often, this is unnecessary and will not increase expected life span. Importantly, the benefits of a bypass can often be achieved with improvements in lifestyle and nutritional medicine. The general rule is to avoid unnecessary surgery; here, we use a bypass as a specific example.

The procedure known as a coronary artery bypass graft is often shortened to CABG, pronounced "cabbage." This description is apt. In open heart surgery, the patient is placed on a heart and lung bypass pump. This operation often results in damage to the brain, called post-perfusion syndrome and colloquially described as "pump-head." So, having a cabbage may turn you into a pump-head. The name is misleading, however, as the problem is not caused by the pump.

Basically, the surgery releases lumps of fat, clots, calcified tissue, and other detritus from the damaged arteries. These enter the bloodstream and travel to the brain, causing multiple mini-strokes. As a result, the patient often suffers from shortened concentration, slower thinking and motor control, and poor short-term memory.[18] Fortunately, the brain has great flexibility and inbuilt redundancy. In the weeks following the bypass, the functions of cells in the damaged regions of the brain are taken over by other brain tissue. As recovery continues, many patients and relatives may not notice the difference.

Heart bypass operations are popular and the significance of the damage to the brain is disputed.[19] However, the use of the term *pump-head* suggests it is a common observation among medical staff. If considering such surgery, ask:

- Will the surgery extend your life?

- Is it being proposed merely to relieve symptoms?

- What benefit can you expect?

- What are the complications and risks?

- Are there other noninvasive alternatives, such as medication?

If you are told that you must have bypass surgery, get a second opinion from a cardiologist, not a surgeon, and ask about minimally invasive surgery. If you decide to go ahead, high-dose antioxidants, such as R-alpha-lipoic acid, melatonin, and vitamins C and E may help prevent damage to your brain.

Almost inevitably, a patient will have strokes during bypass surgery. However, their impact can vary: instead of the mini-strokes, causing pump-head, one or more large blockages may occur in the brain, causing a major stroke.[20] Even with good surgeons, brain complications are far too common. Acute brain disorder (encephalopathy) occurs in about one operation in ten. Clear stroke is less common, but hits about 3 percent of patients. Large strokes may cause death, paralysis, and other obvious problems. Many smaller strokes may cause cognitive deficit (loss of memory and ability to think clearly). If the patient is lucky, they may have fewer small strokes and a large cognitive capacity—clever people may simply be a little less clever, but still not quite what they were before the operation.

In addition to pump-head, there are a large number of specific complications. The bony sternum, which joins the ribs down the midline of the chest, may not heal properly after being cut open. A heart attack can occur if the graft fails, an air bubble is introduced, or there is insufficient blood flow through the transplanted vessels. The graft may close up because of the underlying atherosclerosis, causing a return of angina or heart attack. The kidneys may fail, and the operation is likely to be painful.

Unless your surgery is critically urgent to save your life, you could elect to try a change in diet and to take nutritional supplements. We hope it is unnecessary to suggest stopping smoking. You would need to build up to at least 10,000 mg of vitamin C, spread throughout the day. Ideally, this intake should include some liposomal vitamin C. In addition, you could consider high intakes of mixed tocotrienols (a form of vitamin E), R-alpha-lipoic acid, glucosamine and chondroitin, magnesium chloride, vitamin D_3, and a B-vitamin complex. It is possible to prevent heart disease by changing the diet and the evidence suggests that some supplements and a change in lifestyle can stabilize or even reverse the condition.

It is important to think critically about a CABG before the operation. You may not have the capacity afterward.

cury, which is toxic and can cause brain injury,[17] into vaccines, especially for young children. The choice of having or not having a vaccination should be with the patient.

If the doctor agrees to your position statements, then you are in business. If not, keep looking. Be prepared to spend some time on this initial selection process—it is important to choose the right doctor for you.

RATIONAL PATIENTS

A rational patient is one that lowers their risk of harm. A first principle of game theory is to avoid the maximum cost. In buying a house or car, you negotiate to save money. For a hospital patient, avoiding the maximum cost means making sure you come out alive. Patients can avoid risk of death or crippling debilitation by checking every procedure that is suggested. If you are considering surgery, for example, you might ask the following kinds of questions:

- Do I really need this operation?

- Is the surgery urgent, for example, acute appendicitis or a major aneurism?

- Is there an acceptable conservative treatment?

- What specific benefits will I achieve?

- Heart bypass operations do not usually extend life expectancy, so what is the advantage of having one?

- Will a nose job really change my life?

- Many babies will be born without an elective cesarean, so is there any reason to have one?

- How many times has the surgeon/hospital performed this operation?

- What is the success rate and what does the hospital regard as a success?

- Will I suffer harm?

- All surgery is dangerous—what are the critical dangers of this operation?

- Will I become infected?

- What proportion of patients undergoing this operation in the hospital become infected?

- What happens if I get an antibiotic-resistant bacterial infection?

- How many patients get antibiotic-resistant bacterial infections in this hospital?

This list is by no means exhaustive; there are many possible questions, so concentrate on the major risks. With surgery, the risks associated with anesthetics, DVT, and infections can dominate.

MEDICAL SCREENING

Each screening suggestion from your doctor is likely to start a negotiation. Recently, Dr. Hickey received a letter from the local health center offering an appointment for a health screening. Apparently, the U.K. National Health Service (NHS) was offering tests to all people between the ages of forty and seventy-four who did not have an established risk of heart disease or stroke. The aim of the test was to record a series of risk factors, such as smoking, obesity, poor diet, and so on. The individual risks would be added to determine an overall risk factor and those the test determined to be at high risk would be medicated.

Could this health check initiative be little more than a way of increasing drug sales? There are about 60 million people in the U.K., and 15 million are in this age group. The people for whom such screening is least appropriate are those with no known cardiovascular disease—exactly the group targeted by this initiative. Suppose we assume the test is 90 percent accurate at indicating a clinical problem or good health, which is being generous. This means that 10 percent of healthy people (those not at specific risk) will fail the test. Consequently, 1.5 million people will receive medication from which they will not benefit, but will still suffer the risk of side effects.

The figures necessary for a patient or a doctor to assess the validity of the tests were not published on the NHS website about the health check. So, it was not possible to decide if the screening would be helpful. When asked for specific figures for the tests accuracy, the government's customer service center did not give direct answers. However, they did provide the number of people who were expected to benefit: they predicted that, as a result of the initiative, 1,600 people would not have heart attacks or strokes in a year, and 650 lives might be saved. This seems impressive, until you consider that 15 million people were likely to be tested. So, the chance of benefiting from the test by not having heart disease or stroke is small, approximately one in a thousand. Your risk of not dying is lowered by only 0.004 percent.

Given the information provided, a rational healthy individual would not have the test. Even in a socialized medical system, there is a cost for the "free" test. First, the person taking the test needs to attend the clinic, after fasting overnight, and take a urine sample with them. The claimed minor reduction in risk might be worth this cost. However, to achieve this benefit, the patients who fail the test will need to take drugs for the rest of their lives. So, this small lowering of risk from cardiovascular disease may incur the cost of thirty years' worth of prescriptions and taking one or more drugs each day. As a result of this health screening, some unfortunate people are likely to end up with an unnecessary heart bypass operation. The risks of side effects from the drugs alone are likely to outweigh the small chance of benefit.

Alternative to Cardiovascular Screening

The rational alternative is to have health checks only when you have a reason for thinking you may have a specific problem. Of course, a rational person would take preventive measures to avoid having such a problem by making sure his or her diet is not dominated by junk food, but by eating right and taking supplements. To avoid heart attack and stroke, you can take some specific dietary measures:

1. Avoid sugar—Remove fructose and high-fructose corn syrup from your diet. Fructose is a "sweet poison" and is found in common table sugar as sucrose, which is a combination of glucose and fructose. Similarly, as the name suggests, it is found in high-fructose corn syrup. Glucose is less sweet than fructose and is relatively benign. The toxicity of fructose leads to obesity, type 2 diabetes, high blood cholesterol, and so on. In other words, most of the symptoms addressed in the NHS health check could be reversed by substituting glucose for normal sugar (sucrose), avoiding processed foods (which contain high-fructose corn syrup), and cutting out fruit juices. We are aware that fruit juice is normally considered a health drink but this may be outweighed by the high levels of available fructose.

2. Take supplements—Start with the following program:

- Vitamin C (3,000 mg a day or more, in divided doses)
- Vitamin E (800–1,600 IU a day as natural mixed tocopherols or 100 mg of mixed natural tocotrienols)
- Vitamin B complex (B100 slow release)
- Magnesium (200–400 mg as magnesium chloride or chelated magnesium)
- Fish oil (3,000–5,000 mg)
- A daily multivitamin and mineral

Cardiovascular disease, leading to heart attack or stroke, may simply be a result of chronic nutritional deficiency. It may be possible to prevent or even reverse atherosclerosis and related diseases by taking nutritional supplements. However, these claims have not been tested in randomized clinical trials in humans. So, the rational question to ask is whether investing in these supplements will beat the 0.004 percent reduction in risk provided by the above medical screening and intervention. The authors estimate the probability that nutritional supplements can completely prevent cardiovascular disease as high. Some readers may consider the probability is lower, but we suspect that even the staunchest critics will produce a probability greater than four thousandths of a percent. The associated financial cost is the price paid for good-quality supplements, minus the cost of the drugs you might otherwise be taking. Health benefits of taking supplements rather than drugs include avoiding the drugs' side effects. Supplements themselves have little in the way of negative side effects, but they do have "side benefits," including the possibility of preventing cancer[21] and Alzheimer's disease,[22] along with widespread health benefits.

Dr. Hickey's negotiation for the health check was short. He simply read the leaflets provided and e-mailed the government with a list of questions. The information provided was insufficient to estimate the potential value of the test. The medical establishment was clearly not geared up to provide a response which would allow a patient or doctor even to check the benefits and risks associated with the tests. Looking at this particular health screening initiative using game theory shows that the government was not even providing minimal data. In this negotiation, the government request that he agree to the test was declined as inappropriate and irrational.

RULES FOR NEGOTIATION

Despite the importance of negotiation in our daily lives, we are not taught this skill in school. Negotiation is not an innate attribute, a skill that some people have and others do not; it is a pattern of behavior that can be learned. Most people do not know how to negotiate effectively and many do not even try, inhibited by fear.[23] Such apprehension is even greater for a layperson discussing their health with a highly trained physician.

Some people, such as business managers and salespeople, have an advantage over the physician in discussing possible treatments because they are used to negotiating deals. They weigh the benefits of a deal against its costs on a daily, or even hourly, basis. Others, such as teachers and social workers, have years of experience negotiating with difficult teenagers. If such people inform themselves about their specific diagnosis, they may find it relatively easy to discuss their treatment.

Lawyers are a particular case in which the balance of power can rest with the patient. Physicians are aware that their role in treating disease involves difficult cost-benefit choices. Mistakes are common and any error could result in legal action. Doctors may tread very carefully if the patient or a close family member is a lawyer. However, lawyers need to be careful not to push too hard: if they act in a threatening way, they may receive suboptimal, dangerous, or expensive treatment. If a doctor is scared that her actions may be monitored, she could opt for defensive treatments. In this context, a doctor's rational response would be to protect herself by initiating a large number of diagnostic tests, many of which, such as x-rays or biopsies, might have damaging effects. She may request a costly second opinion to spread the risk. Furthermore, a physician under legal scrutiny would tend not to deviate from standard, conventional treatment. Potentially life-saving surgery might be rejected, for example, based on the risk of complications. When the risks of treatment apply legally to the doctor, as well as medically to the patient, the physician is likely to choose an overly conservative option.

We can compare this situation to eating in restaurants. A difficult customer might be wise to complain and annoy the staff after the meal is finished. We have often heard stories of chefs and waiters spitting in the food of critical customers who made the mistake of complaining too early. In any negotiation, it is essential to consider the position and response of your opponent and adjust your behavior accordingly. Do not threaten legal action, as the response might be directly detrimental to you.

A negotiation occurs whenever you want something from someone else, or they want something from you.[24] All meetings between medical professionals and patients involve negotiation.[25] Fortunately, the rules for successful negotiation have been studied and can be taught. Here, we outline a basic approach, but remember that negotiation is a skill and requires practice.

Before You Visit the Doctor

You should prepare well before visiting a doctor, clinic, or hospital. Your preparation is an essential part of taking and keeping control of your own health. The period before you visit your health-care worker is called the pre-bargaining phase of the negotiation. You need a clear reason for your visit, such as symptoms. Remember that health checks and tests are usually valuable only if you have a specific reason for concern. Make sure you are well prepared by having an aim—some benefit you want to achieve.

Plan Ahead

A critical factor in your negotiation is planning and preparation. Plan your negotiation at an early stage. Decide what you want and consider what you might do if the doctor refuses. You may try to persuade the physician or, alternatively, if seeking private medical care, you could seek a more cooperative medical professional.

Think about how you are going to communicate. Will you have more chance of getting what you want by first talking to the nurse or physician's assistant? You might be able to get information on the hospital's current practices over the telephone. You may ask your family physician to write a supportive letter for your use in the hospital. For those taking supplements, we recommend a "this patient takes vitamins" letter. Even in adulthood, a note from the doctor still carries weight.

Another factor is cost: what is the maximum you can afford for treatment? Will this cover the associated costs? If you can afford the treatment, will the benefit be worth more to you than the cost?

In the event of a complete refusal to cooperate, it may be possible to make small concessions, provided they are reciprocated. For example, a patient might agree to have the operation, provided she is allowed to take her vitamin supplements while in hospital. Any physician that refuses should be asked for a full explanation as to why. One elderly woman we know was in hospital and the staff attempted to take away her vitamins. At ninety years of age, she faced them down, saying: "These supplements are my personal property. You may not take them. If you do, you are stealing from me." They backed off, and she had the procedure.

Gather Information

Gathering information about your health problem is essential. If you have a confirmed diagnosis, find out about the disease and its treatments. Take particular care to find out about the side effects of any drug or therapy. With the advent of Internet search engines, such as Google, medical information has become widely available. Generally, you have access to the same data as your doctors. You will quickly find the authorized sites such as Medscape, but make sure you include sites on nutrition and alternative medicine. If you are not familiar with computers or medical terms, get a friend to help. That young geeky nephew who always seems to be playing computer games has a use. You are aiming to achieve the most benefit (restored health) for the minimum cost, including physical costs such as side effects. Do not be fooled by the common "insurance pays for it." Danger for free is no benefit. Before attending any consultation meetings, be sure you know what the main issues are.

If you are not sure what is ailing you, get background information. Try searching for your symptoms on the Internet.[26] The result might not be an accurate single diagnosis but it may give you an idea of the possibilities. You can generally get what the physicians call a differential diagnosis—the range of possible problems. Don't get carried away, though, or develop the "medical students' disease" (hypochondriasis), worrying that you have every disease you have read about.

When looking up diseases, don't worry if all the symptoms seem to fit your case. A lump in the breast may be cancer, but there are several other less-scary possibilities. Don't agonize until you have a doctor's definite diagnosis. Get one. A solid diagnosis is one of the main benefits of conventional medicine; background information helps you understand the implications.

When you look up your ailment online, use respected sites, such as the *Merck Manual* Medical Library. There are a large number of websites, though few provide reliable information. Conventional sources are preferable for diagnosis and information about disease symptoms. However, this reliability does not always extend to prevention or treatment. Subtle, hidden promotions from the medical industries contaminate conventional information sources. It is useful, however, to learn what the conventional approach has to offer for your illness. When you have the basic information and a solid diagnosis, look at some of the orthomolecular and related websites for natural alternatives.

When your physician suggests a treatment, you need to know the risks and benefits involved. If you have not researched the particular treatment, such as the incidence and severity of side effects, be sure to ask. You should always look up any drug that you are offered before taking it. You need to know the probability that the treatment will be effective: if it only helps one in ten people, you may not want to try that particular therapy. Also, you need to establish whether the drug will be curative or will merely reduce your symptoms to some degree. This is especially the case if the drug has a long list of side effects. Just as you need to know the chance of the drug being effective, it is important to know the risk of side effects. If your doctor cannot provide this information, then find it yourself. Pharmaceutical websites provide extensive lists of side effects, presumably to cover themselves against future litigation.

Set Goals and Expectations

Specify your goals. What do you want to achieve? Are your expectations realistic? Decide the minimum result you would find acceptable, and refuse to accept less. Despite this, remember that half a pie is better than none. Your doctor is not likely to agree to every request. In some cases, there may be genuine concerns. High-dose vitamin therapy may sometimes conflict with some procedures or drugs. But that is not sufficient reason for hospital patients to stop all supplement intakes. If hospital staff want supplement intake halted, make sure you find out exactly why. Which individual supplement is the problem? Ask your doctor. In some cases, a refusal will be in your interests, and a good doctor will be able to provide specific reasons for refusal. A poor doctor may rely on authoritarian arguments and will not be able to give a reasoned explanation based on data.

If your doctor is too busy to provide specific evidence, then the doctor is too busy for you. Get a second opinion.

Before you begin a negotiation, you need to consider your Best Alternative to a Negotiated Agreement (BATNA). The BATNA is the action you will take if the hospital or doctor refuses your requests. Often, the most powerful leverage in a negotiation is the ability to walk away. In many cases, you can find another hospital or doctor; with private medicine, this will lower your health provider's income. If enough patients walk away, their behavior will change or they go out of business. In socialized medicine, such as in the U.K., telling the health-care provider that you find their service inadequate may only affect their reputation.

In some cases, such as emergency surgery, there is no BATNA. You need the doctor's help immediately, and there is no time for negotiation. Fortunately, emergency treatment is where conventional medicine provides its greatest benefit. However, starting nutritional supplementation as soon as possible after surgery may hasten recovery. As soon as the acute emergency is over, patients need to be willing to re-negotiate their treatment.

Establish Rapport

You should aim to build an effective relationship with hospital staff. To this end, it is a good idea to engage the physician in conversation early on in your meetings. Is his or her demeanor friendly and open? You need to find out if the doctor is likely to be willing to cooperate with your needs or will he or she be unnecessarily authoritative. If the doctor is uncooperative and unhelpful, consider choosing an alternative physician.

Consider the doctor's perspective. Most physicians are legally bound and professionally constrained. If you had trained for ten years, how would you react to a know-it-all patient who began to dictate terms in your office? Avoid backing your doctor into a corner. One approach you can use is to introduce materials written by other physicians who treat naturally—journal papers, published treatment plans (protocols), excerpts from books, and highlighted articles. If a reputable doctor uses a natural approach, it may be easier for your doctor to try it with you. Ask for a "therapeutic trial" as the doctor may be willing to see if the proposed therapy has any benefit.

Never mention the words *legal* or *sue* in your discussions. Doctors are genuinely concerned that they could be the subject of legal actions. They are performing a difficult service and are responsible for the good health of their patients. Even the mention of legal action may deter the doctor from treating you. Remember, most doctors are helpful, intelligent, and caring. Threat of litigation will not make them any more so.

Your primary objective in the initial consultation could be to inform your doctor that you are a reasonable, intelligent person, and that your goal is to get back to excellent health. You want to achieve the best possible outcome, without taking unnecessary risks, and understand that you will need to access the doctor's expertise to help achieve your goal. Any reasonable physician would welcome such a patient.

Consider Costs

There is no such thing as a free lunch. Every negotiation has associated costs. There are obvious costs, such as payment for private medical care. In financial terms, popular wisdom suggests you get what you pay for. However, the most expensive specialist may not be the best. One leading surgeon had a reputation for excellence. As a result, he was wealthy but his waiting list was too long and getting him down—he wanted to shorten it and do less work. He decided that increasing his prices should solve the problem, so he doubled them. Ironically, far from cutting his workload, the number of patients requesting his services increased dramatically. Clearly, the surgeon was just as competent before he raised his prices, but his new patients apparently thought that expensive means better. It doesn't—it just means the specialist is making a lot of money. Don't be one of those people who make medical decisions based on inappropriate financial criteria.

There are other kinds of costs. For example, a protracted negotiation during which you upset your doctor could result in delayed treatment, leading to the cost of physical deterioration. The side effects of any treatments are costs, which should be weighed against the potential for improving your condition. We have known numerous patients on so many drugs that it was impossible to tell whether their symptoms were a natural illness or resulted from interactions between their medications.

Consider any surgery carefully. While a particular operation may be essential, increasingly surgery is becoming elective, a lifestyle choice. Before you commit to that nose job or tummy tuck, make sure you are aware of the costs and possible risks. Is trading a flabby tummy for a large, ugly scar line and thousands of dollars really a good decision? Ask yourself what else you could do with the money. Perhaps booking some gym sessions in preparation for a Caribbean holiday could make you happier?

Judge Based on the Merits

Do what works. Always make sure the negotiation is based on merit and avoid letting your emotions drive the process. Illness and treatment are clearly emotive topics, but the more the discussion is based on the merits of the case, the more likely is a satisfactory outcome. When discussing the merits of different courses of action, it is helpful to remember that, in most negotiations, there is a range of fair or acceptable outcomes.[27] The aim is to find an outcome that is optimal for your health, while maintaining a satisfactory relationship with the hospital and its representatives.

You need to ask what treatment options are available. A simple list of possible treatments is not enough—you need sufficient information to enable you make an informed decision. If the list of options does not include your preferred choice, ask about the possibility. For example, a cancer patient offered surgery and chemotherapy, with the alternative of radiotherapy, might ask about nutritional therapy or intravenous vitamin C. The doctor should not dismiss such possibilities but should provide a reasonable and rational justification of his or her recommendations. If you are given a plausible medical reason why you should not use vitamins, be bold and ask for references to the scientific papers from which this was determined.

Given that you have established a level of rapport with the doctor, it is important to decide whether to suggest an option, such as vitamin therapy, or wait and see what the physician proposes. If you suggest an option and the physician states that it is inappropriate, it is the physician's duty to explain the reasons. We keep repeating this because it is important, and you might have to press even for critical information. While the doctor may have specialist education and understanding, you are the patient and the issue is your health; in some cases, your life is at risk. So, the physician has a responsibility to explain the reasons for his decisions and you have an equal responsibility to show respect and consider the evidence provided. Be a good listener, but not a slavish subject.

If the physician suggests a treatment, ask about its effectiveness and possible side effects. How likely is it that the treatment will restore you to health? How frequent are the side effects and how severe might they be? What is the likely outcome if you decline the treatment? If patients do not know the side effects of medications they are taking, they may misinterpret them as a new illness.

When Beta is the Better Format

A classic negotiating scenario, used in business schools, separates the students into two groups, Alpha and Beta. Those in the Alpha group are asked to behave like go-getting business types, negotiating aggressively for the best result. They are individual, impatient, and direct. The members of the Beta group are told to be polite, smile a lot, and never use the word "no." Betas are formal, patient, and indirect. They are deferential to their group's authority and unable to make a decision that does not involve the whole group. Almost invariably, and much to the surprise of the students, the Beta approach is more successful.

Similarly, a Beta approach may be useful in negotiating your health with a physician, as it avoids confrontation without conceding important points. In the business school scenario, Alpha and Beta teams are asked to compete on a specific deal. The Alphas typically make demands and the Betas respond "yes," "maybe," or "we'll have to check and get back to you on that." Typically, the Alphas think that they are winning until close to the end, but they are eventually beaten down, disillusioned by repeated failure to close the deals. One of the reasons for the Betas' success may be the time factor: Alphas tend to be in a hurry, whereas Betas take time to go back to base and consult with the rest of their team. Being short of time is a weakness.

You need time to make sure that you understand the issues. Are you convinced that the proposed treatment will restore you to good health? Is the solution the best option available? What will be the outcome if you do not have the treatment? Is it worth getting a second opinion? What does your local pharmacist think about the drug? If you are unsure about the doctor's proposed treatment, take your time. And so you know you have the time, ask a doctor how long the issue could safely wait. Weeks? Months? Don't be afraid to say you need extra time to think about it. It is a big decision, so consider your options carefully.

Employ a Principal?

In negotiation, a "principal" is a third party with influence or, perhaps, the final decision maker. For example, a small computer company, in Italy, had only one employee. When negotiating contracts, the employee said he had to put all options to his financial director, Mr. Black. Unknown to his negotiating partners, the financial director was a small black terrier! True to his word, he would put the proposal to his dog before returning to the negotiation. "Mr. Black indicates these prices are not justifiable in the current financial circumstances. Is there anything you can do on the price?" The approach was highly effective in negotiating beneficial deals, which illustrates the power of a principal or higher authority.

Applying this method, you might, if you have medical insurance, discuss your options with company representatives before going to see the physician. Not only will you know what will be covered, if the insurance representatives support your approach to treatment, they may provide additional leverage for your suggestions. A layperson negotiating with a doctor is often at a disadvantage because of perceived differences in status and education. You can also use this in reverse: if you are not happy with the proposed treatment, you might tell the physician that you wish to discuss the options with your representative from the insurance company.

Win-Win

Doctors sometimes have odd ideas about medicine. Seeing as many bodies as they do, they can forget that this particular body is yours; your precious health is on the line. You would not expect to take your automobile to a garage for an oil change and then be told that they had decided (unilaterally) to recondition the engine. The mechanic's role is as a professional, providing a service. He has a responsibility to provide advice and technical skill in order to ensure the automobile is an effective, reliable, and safe means of transport. Similarly, the doctor provides a service to the patient. In the doctor's case, the role is to help the patient achieve relief from pain and discomfort, together with freedom from illness. The role extends to helping achieve the optimal physical, mental, and emotional health. In that role, doctors have a duty to make sure patients are satisfied with the treatment.

A win-lose solution is a bad outcome to a negotiation. In particular, you do not want your doctors to feel aggrieved—they might one day wear masks and hold your life in their gloved hands. The result should be satisfactory to all the parties. While you should always negotiate on merit, do not neglect the emotional and other interests of those involved.

Closure

The negotiation is not over until you have achieved a resolution. You may not achieve all your aims, but you should cease negotiating when you are at least satisfied by the outcome. "Satisficing" means achieving a satisfactory outcome, not necessarily the best possible solution. The aim is to achieve a mutually acceptable compromise. If you are dissatisfied with the proposed treatment, there are several options. You can engage the current doctor in further negotiations, explaining that the available options are unappealing or too expensive. You could ask for a second opinion. If you are paying for the treatment, you are free to take your business elsewhere. Look for possible compromises, but don't suggest them, unless the negotiation has reached an impasse.

Stacking the Deck in Your Favor

Make it easy for your doctor by staying healthy. Eating well, not smoking, and avoiding excessive alcohol will show that you take your health seriously. Show that you take care of yourself and expect similar consideration from your physician. Present your doctor with a positive approach to health, just as you might brush your teeth before visiting the dentist.

If you are unconvinced about a proposed therapy, use the "suggestive selling" technique. Suggest a natural alternative to the medical treatment you may be offered. If you are not successful, then, instead of an either-or choice, suggest "both." Know what benefits you want to achieve and see that you get them with minimum risk.

If possible, avoid taking several different drugs, which is known as polypharmacy. Each drug has side effects; if you take two drugs, they can interact. So, you have a three-fold potential risk of side-effects: one set of side effects from each drug and one from the drug interactions. The more drugs you take, the greater the potential for side effects. The number of possible drug interactions also increases rapidly and these interactions are not well understood.

Look up each surgical procedure or medicine you are offered. If you are unsure about doing this yourself, ask someone with an interest in the area to do it. Always ask your pharmacist about a prescribed drug and its side effects. Find out for yourself if there is really a problem with supplementation. It is rare for a vitamin to interfere with a prescription drug. Information about prescription drugs can be found in a number of books, such as the *Physicians' Desk Reference*[28] or the *British National Formulary*.[29] Ask at your local library for sources of information or use the Internet wisely. The necessary information specific for a particular drug should also be contained on its package inserts. Do not assume that your doctor or nurse knows drug interactions for all the available drugs.

Listen for phrases that suggest an open-minded physician:

- "Vitamins aren't likely to do you any harm."

- "I myself take a daily vitamin tablet."

- "I've heard of more and more people doing this."

- "I attended a seminar on this recently."

- "Since it is unlikely to do any harm, let's try it."

- "Let me know how this works out for you."

- "I told my other patients about it."

Doctors love to be told that "their" therapy is successful, so provide your doctor with feedback. Medicine will refocus efforts on nutrition and disease prevention when it becomes apparent to physicians that patients need and request it. It is equally important to let the doctor know when a nutritional intervention is ineffective. If appropriate, tell the doctor that the therapy has worked and you are feeling great. You are likely to be rewarded with, "Whatever you are doing, keep doing it." That is the sweet sound of self-reliant success.

WMD

Ultimately, you could invoke your WMD—weapon of medical destruction— and bring in a lawyer. However, do not make idle threats. We do not support the widespread increase in legal action against the medical profession. Its main actions are to profit lawyers and increase medical costs. However, everyone entering the hospital should have the contact details of a legal representative. Hospitals are dangerous places and a lawyer can be your ultimate weapon. Legal action is always a last possible resort and must be avoided if there is any reasonable alternative. Involving lawyers, or even mentioning them, may prevent doctors from providing you with the best care. As mentioned previously, you may be subjected to excessive diagnostic testing and procedures, as the physicians cover their actions with defensive medicine. Once you have invoked legal action, health care may be more difficult to find. Even excellent doctors do not want patients who encourage legal challenge of their best efforts.

Medical doctors do a difficult job under challenging circumstances with a constantly changing knowledge base. Unless conditions are extreme and patients have suffered gross neglect or life-threatening incompetence, simply side-step inept or prejudiced doctors. Take control of your life and manage your case yourself. Avoid the transferring of responsibility from one flawed profession (doctors) to another (lawyers), and having to pay for both.

CHAPTER 7

Take Charge of Your Health Care

"The doctor of the future will give no medicine,
but will instruct his patient in the care of the human frame,
in diet, and in the cause and prevention of disease."
—Thomas Alva Edison (1847–1931)

It is a cornerstone of corporate medicine that doctors are needed in order for people to make rational decisions about their health. Doctors, it is assumed, have the training and information needed for such life-and-death decisions and ordinary people do not. While it is true that patients suffering from dementia may need help with even day-to-day decisions, a motivated intelligent adult is at little or no disadvantage compared to a physician. Medical doctors have no special access to privileged information and no specialist training in rational decision making. Perhaps it is time doctors respected the primary authority of the patient.

GET THE CORRECT DIAGNOSIS

When you are ill, the first critical focus is to find out what is wrong with you. While there are some general ways of helping the healing process, most treatments depend on the specific diagnosis; there is no point in giving an inappropriate treatment. One of the main functions of doctors is to make a diagnosis, which provides information, suggesting possible treatments and the likely outcome.

To be useful, the diagnosis must be accurate. Errors at this stage may be compounded if incorrect treatment is given that causes the patient increased harm or endangers their life. As a senior surgeon once told us, diagnosis is more of an art than a science: it depends upon clinical judg-

147

ment. Medicine is not a science and is more accurately described as a craft or technology. Clinical decisions have no unique properties and are well explained by the decision sciences. Unfortunately, a doctor's judgment is often subjective. They might do well to learn some simple decision-science techniques and to use computer aids.[1] Medical diagnosis may be described as an art, but it has a basis in science and could easily be improved.

Inappropriate decisions cause errors. Strangely, medical errors are often not a major concern for either patients or doctors, though this may simply reflect ignorance of the facts. Dr. Robert Blendon and colleagues did a national survey of 831 physicians, who responded to mailed questionnaires. About one-third of the physicians (35 percent) reported medical errors. The researchers compared this result with random telephone interviews with 1,207 members of the public. A large proportion of the public (42 percent) reported medical errors in their family's care.[2] A similar study of 2,201 adults supported these observations.[3] Of these, 35 percent reported that their immediate family had suffered a medical error in the previous five years. Half of the errors were misdiagnoses and 35 percent of these produced permanent harm or even death. Over twice as many adults (55 percent) were concerned about outpatient diagnoses, compared with those provided in a hospital (23 percent). Similar worries about the appropriateness of treatment (38 percent) and misdiagnosis (22 percent) were found in patients receiving emergency treatment.[4] Somehow despite this widespread experience, medicine is often considered caring and effective.

Accurate Methods of Diagnosis

Some methods of diagnosis are less subjective and likely to produce accurate results. Pathology and laboratory examination of specimens should give reproducible results. Radiology, which involves recognizing magnetic resonance, x-ray, or ultrasound images, is also reasonably accurate.[5] For these approaches, typical error rates are reported to vary between two and five misdiagnoses per 100 patients. With surgical pathology specimens, a second opinion resulted in only 86 altered diagnoses in 6,171 patients, suggesting reasonable consistency.[6] However, these low error rates depend on the skill and interpretation of medical specialists; when radiographs are interpreted by physicians in an emergency department, from 16 percent to 35 percent were incorrect.[7] As we have described earlier, medical tests are typically not accurate enough to be considered reliable. Always ask for a second test, particularly if the doctor suggests you have an unexpected result.

Gerd Gigerenzer, psychologist and Director of the Max Planck Institute for Human Development, in Berlin, has investigated medical diagnosis and decision making. He came to the conclusion that physicians are often unable to interpret the results of diagnostic tests.[8] Dr. Gigerenzer found that simple methods, such as representing probabilities as fractions, such as 23 people in 100 rather than a probability of 0.23, greatly improved doctors' ability to understand the meaning of basic diagnostic results.[9] Unfortunately, doctors are given almost no training in such statistics. Moreover, there is a trend in medicine to represent results in terms of percentages and relative risks, which simply confuse the reader, whether medically trained or not. Even when tests provide definitive results, doctors may misunderstand their implications.

Error-Prone Diagnoses

Direct clinical observation can provide robust results but, often, such evidence is vague. The proportion of errors in clinical diagnoses is higher than with experimental or radiographic data. In British hospitals, according to one study, 6 percent of the admission diagnoses were found to be in error.[10] Almost 11 percent of hospital patients in Greater London had adverse events, more than half of which could have been prevented. Of these patients, less than one-fifth of the adverse events were caused by surgery or invasive procedures; more than half were caused by errors on the wards. Diagnoses by inexperienced clinicians, poor records, insufficient communication, inadequate consultant support, and inappropriate assessment before discharge were identified as contributory factors.

The current popularity of so-called evidence-based medicine (EBM) means that doctors are guided in their practice of diagnosis and treatment by the results of large clinical trials. Unfortunately, large-scale trials are next to useless in this respect. The idea that you can use the statistics of groups to predict the response in an individual is a fallacy. Gamblers know this well, often to their regret. Indeed, such error even has a scientific name—the *ecological fallacy*. To take an extreme example of this error, in human beings, the average number of ovaries and testicles across the population is one of each! Clearly, a surgeon operating on a randomly selected individual would be unlikely to find this particular arrangement of organs. In this case, the group is really two groups—males and females —so the average is nonsensical. However, human anatomy and physiology are biologically individual, so it is improbable that a doctor will ever meet an "average" patient.[11] Serious mistakes occur when group averages are attributed to an individual.

Diagnoses made in emergency departments are particularly difficult, as staff members operate a high patient load under time constraints. Emergency doctors are often subject to stress and uncertainty, which can lead to diagnostic errors. In addition, emergency medicine often requires complex and rapid decision making concerning life-threatening situations. The rate of misdiagnosis in emergency rooms is variable, but is reported to be from 0.6 percent[12] to 12 percent.[13] The divergence in these figures may simply reflect different definitions of misdiagnosis.

One reason for doctors making so many mistakes in diagnosis and treatment is overconfidence. Too often, a medical doctor seems to want to be thought of as a sort of deity, and many patients are only too happy to oblige. Patients should give doctors the respect that comes with their education and professional standing. However, the converse is also true: doctors should respect patients, who regardless of their education, gender, race, or economic standing, deserve courtesy. Indeed some patients are better educated and of higher standing than their physician. The unwarranted assumption of power may lead physicians to become overconfident, which can result in errors in diagnosis.[14]

MINIMIZE THE RISKS OF MEDICAL SCREENING

Medical tests can be dangerous: they might put you in the hospital. Such repercussions should be considered carefully. Screening tests such as body scanning or mammography are difficult to justify. The tests are simply too inaccurate, given the small chance that a typical subject has the disease. Many doctors do not realize this, thinking that a positive test means that the subject is almost certain to be ill. The broader implication of medical testing is that screening a person in good health is likely to be harmful.

To take an example, let us assume we have a mammogram test for breast cancer that is 90 percent accurate. This means that for ten people who have the illness, nine will have a positive test. At first glance, such a result looks great, as those nine can now have treatment. However, some

"How Long Have I Got?"

On hearing they have malignant cancer, patients often respond with the question "How long have I got, doctor?" In some cases, the doctor will reassure the patient that there are treatments available. In most common adult malignancies, the physician will know that treatments are unlikely to save the patient. Doctors face a dilemma: answering honestly is an admission of failure, but the patient wants an idea of the length of time they have, so they can say goodbye and make arrangements.

"So," said comedian Henny Youngman, "This guy's doctor told him he had six months to live. The guy said he couldn't pay his bill. The doctor gave him another six months." The joke is more apt than it appears. Let's say the doctor gives an opinion, based on ten years' of experience in cancer treatment, that the patient has four to six months to live. The patient then uses this estimate to plan, survives for eight months, and feels lucky for beating the odds. However, the doctor's estimate of life expectancy is likely to be almost useless for any individual case and should probably be ignored, as another illustration of the ecological fallacy.

As an example, biologist and author Stephen Jay Gould was diagnosed in 1982 with mesothelioma.[15] As a scientist, Dr. Gould's response was to ask where the best technical literature on his illness was. The physician told him there was nothing worth reading about the disease. Perhaps she was being kind—on average, half the people with this disease would be dead in only eight months. However, Dr. Gould knew he *might* achieve a much longer life, as some people with the disease live for years. He understood the statistics better than his doctor. In the end, he recovered and survived for twenty years and eventually died of a different (lung) cancer.

In one study, doctors were asked how long 193 patients with Hodgkin's disease, a cancer of white blood cells, would live.[16] Their estimates were essentially random, about as good as taking a number from a hat. Suppose you are fifty and expected to live to age eighty but now have prostate cancer. Picking a random number between fifty and eighty is as accurate as your doctor's estimate. As iconoclastic optimists, we suggest you break the rules and choose age eighty-five. Most people with prostate cancer die with it rather than from it.

Some patients with "terminal" cancer will greatly exceed the doctor's expectations, living a long and gratifyingly productive life. Given a terminal diagnosis, the patient would do well to consider changing their lifestyle. A rational terminal patient, aware of the nature of the disease, would take some specific supplements and change their diet to improve their chances.[17] Yogi Berra was right: "It ain't over 'til it's over."

of the people with positive mammograms may have a form of cancer called ductal carcinoma in situ (DCIS).[18] If left untreated, some women with DCIS will not go on to develop breast cancer. Following the mammogram, DCIS patients may be considered as cancer sufferers; they could have their tumors removed, followed by radiotherapy and, possibly, chemotherapy. They might even be happy, considering themselves the lucky ones because their "cancer" was found early. The doctors benefit too, as their apparent cure rates go up, treatment statistics improve, and they can use the data to support additional screening. However, some of these patients will have been "cured" of a disease they never actually had and, if not for the mammogram, they could have lived their whole lives in blissful, healthy ignorance.

To minimize the risks associated with medical testing, we need to understand how they work. You cannot rely on the expertise of your doctors; many of them are as confused by statistics as the rest of us.

In order for you to make a rational decision, the doctor needs to be able to tell you more than the "accuracy" of the test. A doctor who tells a patient that a test is about 90 percent accurate, or even 99.99 percent accurate, has not conveyed enough information. The patient cannot use this figure to work out whether or not they should have the test. The patient also needs to know the accuracy of the test on people who do not have the disease. So, an important question is, if a subject does not have the illness, what is the likelihood of the test reporting this accurately? To keep things simple, we will assume that the test is also around 90 percent accurate for people who do not have the illness. On hearing this figure, people may feel reassured that the test is useful. After all, if the test only misses one in ten people who have the disease, and misclassifies only one in ten people who do not have it, that is not too bad, is it? We might think it is worth subjecting one person to gratuitous treatments, in order to save another person's life (although the first person might disagree).

Unfortunately, we still do not have enough information to make this decision. In order to decide whether or not a screening test is likely to be beneficial, we also need to know the incidence of the disease in the population. This is the chance that a typical person in the population will get the disease over some period of time. In mammography, for example, we need to know the chance of a typical person developing breast cancer.

Let us use figures published by David Eddy for the accuracy of mammography.[19] As an example, let us suppose that you are a typical, apparently healthy woman and your chance of having breast cancer is one in 1,000. (Men also get breast cancer, but the frequency is lower.) You take a mammographic screening test, which gives a positive result. What is the chance that you actually have breast cancer? The test's accuracy is 92 percent, so most people, including many doctors, would assume this meant a 92 percent chance of having the disease. Fortunately, they are wrong: even if you have a positive result, you are still unlikely to have the disease. If you really did have cancer, there is a 92 percent chance of the disease being picked up. Similarly, if you are healthy, the test will be correct 88 percent of the time. Now—and this is important—remember that the incidence of breast cancer is only one in 1,000. So, for 1,000 people tested, only one will have the disease and have a positive test (at 92 percent accuracy). By contrast, 999 people will not have the disease, of whom 120 (at 88 percent accuracy) will be wrongly diagnosed false-positives. Therefore, if you have a positive test, your result is much more likely to be false than true. Your probability of having the illness with a positive test is only one in 120, or less than 1 percent!

Of course, as a patient with a positive screening result, you are likely to be worried and concerned about having the illness. You will probably be recalled for additional tests. The initial test might be repeated just to be sure. If the result of the second test is positive, you may well be even more worried. However, even after two positive tests, the chance of having cancer is still less than 10 percent, despite the test's 92 percent accuracy. This can be seen in the following way: of the 121 positive results of the first test, on average only one will be correctly diagnosed as having the illness, while 120 healthy people will be misclassified as sick. The chance of an apparently healthy person having the disease after two positive tests is only 7 percent. However, many may consider two positive tests "proof."

Before the test you were apparently healthy and happy. Now, you may be scared enough to go for additional tests and perhaps a surgical biopsy. If this shows abnormal cells (which, if undetected, might never have caused a problem), you could be in for treatment. Conservative treatment might be lumpectomy (removal of the lump), followed by radiation therapy. If you have a more radical surgeon, you might have a radical mastectomy, together with radiation or chemotherapy. Living in fear of a relapse, you are likely to be monitored and frequently rechecked for the next few years. However, you could well have been healthy and likely to remain that way.

Basic Rules for Medical Tests

Ask the physician to explain your individual need for the test. This should include the reason the doctor considers you may have the disease. In an ideal world, the doctor will be able to tell you the test's accuracy, both for those with the disease and for those who are healthy. You would also be told the incidence of the disease in the population and in any high-risk group to which you belong. You also need to know what will happen if the test indicates you may have the disease. Will the follow-up be invasive? Might you receive treatment for a disease you do not actually have?

Staff and students at Harvard Medical School found test results difficult and failed to interpret them properly.[20] They were asked about the meaning of an accurate positive diagnostic test result. The medics had been told that the illness occurred in one person in 1,000. Of those who did not have the illness, 5 percent (50 in 1,000) would test positive. The subjects were asked, what is the chance that a person with a positive result has the disease? About half of the respondents said the probability was 95 percent that such a patient had the illness. This answer is wrong. If 1,000 people took the test, then 51 would be expected to test positive: 50 false-positives and one person with the illness. Of those 51 positive results, only one person was really ill ($1/51 \approx 2$ percent). So, only 2 percent of those with a positive test would have the disease, not 95 percent, as many of the medics believed. Worryingly, the medics who failed this test were from an elite medical school and presumably represent the cream of the profession.

In the real world, the doctor (even a specialist) will not be able to provide you with all this information. A general practitioner is not expected to remember the incidence of every disease and the statistics for all clinical tests. As we have seen, the necessary figures are often difficult to obtain. Despite this, doctors administering screening tests should be able to provide such information. Critically, without this information the test may simply be misleading. You can glean what information the doctor is able to provide and then do further research. Find out about the test. If you do not understand test statistics, find someone who does.

Here are some rules of thumb to help you decide whether or not to be tested.

You should have a diagnostic test:

- If you have good reason to believe you have the disease.

- If you are in a high-risk group. Being in a high-risk group means that the likelihood of your having the disease is greater. This means the test has more value as a positive test might indicate a higher risk of having the illness.

- If you have symptoms. Having relevant symptoms places you in a high-risk group. Something is generating signs of disease, such as breast lumps, and you need to ensure that you are safe.

- If the test is exceedingly accurate. A really accurate test would overcome the problems of diseases with a low incidence. If the test is highly accurate, a patient with a low risk who tests positive will probably have the disease. However, medical tests are performed on biological systems, which are characteristically variable. People also vary, so highly accurate diagnostic tests are rare.

- If the risk is large. Risk includes the likelihood that you have the disease and the magnitude of its consequences. It is pointless having a test if the health cost of the disease is minimal. For example, infection with benign gut bacteria is irrelevant if the bug is naturally present and does no harm.

You should not have the test:

- If you have no reason to believe you are at risk. In this case, a screening test may be counterproductive and ultimately cause you harm.

- If you are not in a high-risk group. Then, you are, by definition, unlikely to have the disease. In this case, the test is unlikely to be accurate, unless you have symptoms.

- If you don't have symptoms. If you do not have symptoms and are not at specific (high) risk of contracting the disease, the test is unlikely to be useful.

- If the test is not accurate. An inaccurate test is useless unless you are at very high risk, have some decidedly specific symptoms, or have a strong reason to believe you have the disease.

- If you receive too little information. You need three pieces of information before you can judge the value of any test: the test accuracy for people who have the illness (also called the incidence of true positives and false negatives); the test accuracy for those do not have the illness (also called the incidence of true negatives and false positives); and the incidence of the disease in the group of people to which you belong. The doctor proposing the test should be able to provide this information.

WHY YOU DON'T NEED
HIGH-TECHNOLOGY MEDICINE

People do not need doctors and high-technology hospitals to maintain good health. Corporate medicine deals with the sick and is little help with disease prevention and promoting good health. Doctors get little training in nutrition at medical school and only rarely embark on independent nutritional studies. Over the years, corporate medicine has acted to inhibit people from taking nutritional supplements or having a good diet. Since the decision, long ago, that they would predominantly target the sick, it may be time for them to stay out of preventive medicine altogether.

It is not clear whether corporate medicine is of overall benefit to patients, even though doctors and hospitals often save lives and prevent disability. We will repeat the caveat that if you are unfortunate enough to break bones or have acute appendicitis, a hospital may save your life. However, there is solid evidence that hospitals also kill and maim. Overall, do hospitals reduce disability and extend people's lives? Obtaining an answer might seem straightforward: if the number of people killed is subtracted from the lives saved, we would have an indication of the overall

Fantasy Surgery

Fantasy surgery is a term that refers to operations carried out to forestall problems that might not occur. A twentieth-century example is the removal of tonsils from children, just in case they might become infected.[21] In 1934, a study in New York found that 610 out of 1,000 children (61 percent) had had their tonsils removed. Doctors then examined about 370 of the remaining children (37 percent), to see whether they required tonsillectomy. They recommended that 45 percent (about 166) of the children should have the operation. This left about 204 "healthy" children, who were presented to other doctors as new patients. The new doctors selected a similar proportion for surgery (46 percent or 94 children), leaving about 110, who had been classified as healthy children twice. These twice-healthy children were then examined by a further set of doctors to see if they needed tonsillectomy, which resulted in only 64 children (of the original group of 1,000) who had not been recommended for the operation. The study ended, apparently, because there were no more physicians to advise the remaining children to have the operation.

George Bernard Shaw would seem to have been correct when he commented, "The test to which all methods of treatment are finally brought is whether they are lucrative (to doctors) or not." As the tonsillectomy example suggests, each time a doctor examines a patient, the patient may risk unnecessary treatment and financial cost.[22] Unless the patient has ominous symptoms, a clinical examination or other test may do more harm than good. This is particularly the case with mass medical screening, which is becoming increasingly common.

utility. The numbers are not published. Currently, there is no convincing evidence that, on average, hospitals benefit the health of society.

The publication of the number of people who were dying as a result of medical interventions has generated concerns about the quality of treatment.[23] In 2004, the U.S. Institute for Health-care Improvement (IHI) responded with the 100,000 Lives Campaign.[24] The Institute approached over 3,000 U.S. hospitals, with the aim of preventing 100,000 unnecessary deaths over eighteen months. They wanted the hospitals to use six interventions that might help protect patients:

- Rapid response teams

- Medication reconciliation

- Prevent central line infections

- Prevent surgical site infections

- Prevent ventilator-associated pneumonia

- Evidence-based care for myocardial infarction

The idea was that by setting a number of lives to be saved, the aims would be clear and results measurable.[25] Eighteen months later, in June 2006, IHI proudly announced that the campaign had far surpassed its goal, as 122,342 lives had been saved.[26] According to their reports, hospitals had responded successfully to the challenge laid down by the campaign.[27] Self-congratulation was the order of the day. One paper even suggested, without a hint of irony, that a new target should be set: a 5 Million Lives Campaign.[28] Admitting that 15 million adverse events occurred in hospitals each year, it was suggested that there were forty to fifty incidents for each 100 hospital admissions.[29] The aim of the new campaign was to lower the number of adverse event deaths by 5 million a year.

Despite these well-publicized campaigns, unnecessary hospital deaths and injuries continue to happen. Even the estimates for the number of lives saved in the 100,000 Lives Campaign were optimistic.[30] There is no reliable evidence to support this claim. In 2009, the Agency for Health-care Research and Quality (AHRQ) provided a check of the figures. They reported a decrease of 23,623 deaths between 2004 and 2006. Using the dates of the campaign, they suggested, only 12,342 lives were saved.[31] The idea of lowering the harm done in hospitals was laudable. Unfortunately, the effort was a failure: people are still being killed and maimed in hospitals.

For millions of years, humans and their ancestors have thrived without doctors and organized medicine. Over the past 2,000 or so years, people survived despite the bloodletting, barbaric operations, and purging that physicians used to think were therapeutic.

Over recent years, corporate medicine has tended to destroy or abuse many of the most effective tools at its disposal. In 200 years, it has essentially failed to improve vaccination beyond its crude beginnings and still injects animal tissue and various viruses, along with the supposedly protective antigen. To this concoction, product developers have added various toxic additives and preservatives, which potentially cause autoimmune disease and neurotoxicity. Hospitals have failed to maintain reasonable standards of hygiene and consequently have acted as breeding grounds for antibiotic-resistant organisms.

The medical professions have abused and overused antibiotics, promoting the development of resistant pathogens. In late 2009, the first case of XXDR TB was found in the U.S., an extremely drug-resistant form of tuberculosis, which is even more dangerous than multi-drug-resistant tuberculosis (MDR TB) and extensively drug-resistant TB (XDR TB). MDR TB is resistant to at least two primary first-line drugs, isoniazid and rifampicin. Modern medicine would do well to remember that diseases such as TB ravaged Western populations a relatively short time ago. It could return. In 2007, there were 9 million new cases and almost 2 million deaths from the illness.[32] Half a million people are estimated to have MDR TB.

In the past, TB was epidemic in Europe, with one in four people dying from the disease. Over time, TB and other infections were defeated largely by changes in lifestyle and improved nutrition. Fortunately, a good immune system can prevent the disease from developing in as many as 90 percent of people.[33] In other words, people can be infected with TB for long periods without harm. The illness breaks through when the body's immune system cannot keep the person healthy.

Drug-resistant TB most often arises when doctors fail to treat it properly or patients do not adhere to the long treatment schedule. Notably, MDR TB spreads from person to person in places where people have compromised or poor immune systems. XXDR TB may be resistant to all first-line and second-line antibiotics. Relying on antibiotics and treatment, rather than an excellent immune system, to protect against pandemic diseases is irrational.

Individuals can support their immune systems and greatly lower their risk of infection by ensuring they are not nutritionally deficient. The key vitamins are C and D_3. Most people do not obtain sufficient amounts of either. In temperate regions, people can manufacture their own high levels of vitamin D when exposed to the summer sunshine. During the winter, however, vitamin D levels drop, which may be the driving factor for the cold and flu season.[34] If you get a cold or the flu every year or two, it is time to reassess your diet and consider vitamin supplements.

THE DOCTOR WITHIN

A classic case report from 1940 concerns a boy with an abnormal craving for salt.[35] His first word was "salt." At one year old, the boy began licking the salt off crackers and eating it directly from the salt shaker. At every opportunity, the boy would eat salt. His parents, concerned at this abnormal behavior, consulted a doctor. The boy was taken to the hospital, where extra salt was not available, and he died. The doctors failed to recognize that the child had a problem with his adrenal glands, causing shortage of the hormones that regulate salt excretion. His body could not retain salt and his hunger for it was a compensation mechanism. The boy needed salt and would go to great lengths to maintain his intake. By restricting his salt, the hospital inadvertently killed him.

It is strange to think that this little boy's body knew more about his nutritional needs than a hospital. Fortunately, the case of the boy who loved salt is an outlier—few people will have such a salt requirement. However, the case demonstrates that human requirements for nutrients can vary widely, a factor that is not taken into account in determining recommended dietary allowances. Sixty years after a hospital killed the little salt boy, medicine still does not accept the variability in need for vitamins and minerals.

Just like humans, animals have specific vitamin and mineral requirements and will seek out sources of nutrients and adjust their diet accordingly. Elephants dig out saltlicks to satisfy their need for minerals, including salt and iodine.[36] In places where the soil is deficient in sodium, termite mounds may be used as saltlicks. Many other animals visit saltlicks and use them to obtain adequate intakes of calcium, magnesium, selenium, sodium, and zinc. Dairy cattle are given saltlicks that are loaded with trace minerals.

While humans retain some ability to select food for the nutrients we require, animals are more effective and even self-medicate.[37] Dogs and jackals often eat grass;[38] there are several explanations for this behavior, but the most likely one is that canines use grass as a medicine for gastrointestinal upsets. Cats also commonly eat grass, presumably for similar medicinal reasons.[39] Baboons in Ethiopia selectively eat balanites fruit when at risk of schistosomiasis, a disease caused by a fluke of fresh-water snails. The fruit contains a powerful drug, diosgenin, which may help protect against infection.[40] Tanzanian chimps use aspilia, which is antibacterial, antifungal, and helps prevent worms. However, the drug is not well absorbed when swallowed. To overcome this, the chimps knead the leaves around their mouths before swallowing, to encourage buccal absorption. Aspilia is important in African traditional medicine as well.[41]

Wild orangutans have been observed using a natural anti-inflammatory.[42] In 2005, Dr. Helen Morrogh-Bernard, of Cambridge University, was studying the great apes in Borneo.[43] She saw an adult female grab leaves from a plant and chew them. Then, taking some of the foamy green spit, the ape applied it to her left arm. Dr. Morrogh-Bernard immediately realized the ape must be applying the leaves as a form of self-medication. The leaves came from commelina, also known as dayflowers, which orangutans do not normally eat. Local people use the plants as a medication: they grind it up and apply it to their skin as an anti-inflammatory treatment for muscular pain and swelling. Other apes also used the leaves as a skin treatment. Dr. Morrogh-Bernard acknowledges the herbal link between the apes and the local people, both of whom use the same treatment, and she speculates that the people may have learned about the drug from the apes.

Animals adjust their behavior, movement, and diet to ensure they have adequate mineral intakes. Modern humans are not so lucky—we consume so much processed and otherwise adulterated food that it confuses our ability to control our diets. An example of this contamination is the widespread introduction of monosodium glutamate (MSG), which is used to make otherwise unpalatable food tastier. At high intakes, MSG is a neurotoxin that kills brain cells and is somewhat addictive.

THE NEW MEDICINE

A new initiative is taking hold in medicine, supported by improvements in communication and collaboration brought about by the Internet. The ramifications may be immense and unforeseeable. Looking back to 1977, Ken Olson, President of Digital Equipment Corporation (then a leading computer company), told the World Future Society in Boston, "There is no reason anyone would want a computer in their home." It is easy to be smug after the event, but few could have predicted the rise of ubiquitous computing and the Internet. Similarly, corporate medicine may have missed the implications of the new technology in their field.

As many people are aware, the World Wide Web has developed a more collaborative technology, commonly called Web 2.0, which facilitates information sharing and cooperation. Health 2.0 and Medicine 2.0 are used by people with an interest in health care, including doctors, scientists, and patients.[44] The aim is to increase participation in health care and medicine through social networking, participation, apomediation, collaboration, and openness.

Most of these terms are self explanatory. Apomediation is when someone filters and interprets the information. An apomediator is anyone with extensive knowledge of the area; an intelligent patient who has researched an illness and produced a website is an apomediator. Apomediators may have no formal qualifications or could be university professors. However, apomediators often have more specialist knowledge than physicians. It seems that the idea of apomediators was not initially considered part of the process. Dean Giustini, a librarian at the University of British Columbia Biomedical Branch, suggested, "An expert [that is, doctor] moderated repository of the knowledge base, in the form of a medical wiki, may be the answer to the world's inequities of information access in medicine if we have the will to create one."[45] Limiting the information to that approved by a physician may have been suggested to placate physicians. However, almost immediately it became apparent that medical knowledge is not the proprietary domain of doctors, nor was it ever so. The new open approach to medicine provides almost endless opportunities for improving health in the future.[46]

TAKING CONTROL OF YOUR HEALTH CARE

Doctors have a vested interest in controlling of your health care. Participative medicine involves patients retaining responsibility for the final decision; the doctor's role should be to provide information and technical expertise. Ultimately, you should decide whether or not surgery is appropriate in your case or if the benefits of a prescribed drug outweigh the risks. The doctor should inform you of the side effects and potential benefits: if a doctor is prescribing a drug, he or she should be able to justify that recommendation.

Naturally, doctors have criticized Health 2.0 and patients' use of the Internet. These tools may be seen as threatening to their status and livelihood. They argue that while doctors might validly use Google to help diagnosis, this does not apply to the general public. The claim is that people who are not qualified physicians might be "less efficient and be less likely to reach a correct diagnosis."[47] Surprisingly, in experimental testing, individual "human experts" get worse results than does a nonspecialist but informed crowd.[48] Moreover, we consider it highly unlikely that a typical M.D. would outperform a well-educated apomediator, although, like the critics of Health 2.0, we have no specific data on this point.

Can you manage your own health care?

This is a strange question, but one that is often asked of patients by doctors and other health-care professionals. Often, the answer is a simple "yes." The management of your health is ultimately your choice. Indeed, the failings of corporate medicine mean that it is essential that people take more responsibility for their own care. If you will not take the trouble to minimize your risk, do not expect the hospital to take such care.

Health is too big a topic for any one person to know it all, and that includes doctors. Most intelligent patients can rapidly learn more about their own condition than a typical general practitioner is likely to know. Read a book or paper, and the words you will read are the same as a physician reads. In fact, you may discover material that your busy doctor has never found or perhaps not investigated in detail. In addition, you can ask your doctor to provide supplementary information or to explain medical terminology or the implications of what you have found. If patients investigated their ailments before they visited the doctor, they would improve the chance of effective treatment and of not being harmed. The doctor should encourage you to participate in your health care.

Is a little knowledge dangerous?

In our experience, some medical professionals are not comfortable with well-informed patients. The patients may be engineers, architects, or research scientists, with at least the intellect and education of a medical consultant. Strangely, physicians expect special treatment and acknowledgment of their status. We have even seen bemused world-famous professors being talked down to as if they were children by low-status hospital staff.

Both doctors and patients are increasingly turning to the Internet for information. However, if the patient asks a question as a result of what he read, a doctor may ask, condescendingly, if he found that out by reading it on the Web. Such an attitude is unprofessional. The patient's efforts should be supported, not discouraged. Plus, the doctor will likely be getting a high proportion of his or her information from the same source.

The increasing availability of knowledge has led to a new initiative called participatory medicine. The Society for Participatory Medicine began in 2009 to extend the work of medical self-care pioneer Tom Ferguson, M.D., who came up with the concept of the "e-patient": an Internet-aware and capable patient who expects to discuss health issues with the doctor. Physicians who refuse to hold such discussions risk damaging the doctor-patient relationship[49] and losing credibility as professionals.

Doctors sometimes warn against the dangers of patients who gather medical information using the Internet, suggesting they may get factually incorrect information, leading to serious harm.[50] There is so much wildly irrational information on the Web, they claim, that patients may be confused and delay going to see their doctor.[51] This appears to be a biased and condescending argument, as intelligent people using the Internet can tell that many sites are rubbish. They are already aware of the need to filter medical data carefully and to discuss it with their physician. The record of harm caused by relying on corporate medicine is the greater problem. Most medical practice is irrational and not based on science, so intelligent patients should check all the information they receive, regardless of whether it comes from the Internet or from their doctor. Both are prone to error.

Isn't a doctor's special province to be the authority on health?

An authority is someone with the power or right to make decisions; "the authority" is an expert whose views are taken as definitive. In the first case, a doctor has power to make decisions about a person's health to the extent permitted by that person; that is why we have consent forms, for example. In the second case, most doctors' opinions are not considered definitive, as medicine is complex and differences of opinion are the norm.

Patients may perceive a doctor as having a level of authority that exceeds his or her knowledge; certain arrogant or insecure doctors may even encourage such perceptions. Although physicians and surgeons have a long period of university and hospital training before they can practice, whole bodies of knowledge in healing are omitted from the curriculum. Even at the point of graduation, doctors can be aware of only a minute fraction of the relevant information. Each year, thousands of research papers are published, so medical practitioners have little or no chance of remaining up to date, especially family doctors, who see patients from many specialist areas.

Participatory medicine recognizes that any doctor's knowledge is necessarily limited and acknowledges the skills of the patient. Suppose a world-famous professor of genetics came down with an hereditary illness. A general practitioner would be very unlikely to have greater knowledge of the disease. In such a case, the geneticist should not refrain from checking the Internet or any other resources in deference to the physician. Even the consultant physician specializing in the disease and its treatment would be wise to respect and listen to this patient. This is an extreme example, but any patient may have the time and motivation to become more of an expert in their own disease than a typical doctor, whose time is spread thin.

In many fields, so-called laypeople have made valuable contributions. Advances in mathematics, science, and medicine have arisen from outside the disciplines, often inspired by people with limited formal education. Famous examples include the mathematician Srinivasa Ramanujan, the physicist George Green, and the milkmaids who told Edward Jenner how to avoid smallpox. Being a patient does not remove your intellect.

Doctors may be authorities in some sense, but that does not prevent Professor Stuart Sutherland using them as examples throughout his book *Irrationality*.[52] Physicians and surgeons are no better (or worse) at making rational decisions than anyone else. To remain healthy, whenever possible, you need to take responsibility for your treatment. There are numerous specialist websites, created by patients and others with a particular interest, which can help you with this aim. These often provide a simple explanation of symptoms, diseases, and treatments. Moreover, the doctor who chides you for researching on the Internet may well be using the same site.

Isn't the science of modern medicine too much for a layperson to learn?

Richard Feynman was the leading physicist of his generation. He defined science as a belief in the ignorance of the experts. He also argued that "if you can't explain something to a first-year student, then you haven't really understood it." Albert Einstein said something similar and both were dealing with aspects of physics, which are acknowledged to be conceptually difficult. Likewise, an able doctor should be capable of explaining your disease or symptoms to you in a straightforward way. If the doctor cannot explain your illness or the treatment, get a second opinion from someone who can. However, ask four different doctors and you may receive four different diagnoses or prescriptions.

Taking charge of decisions about your health seems an awesome responsibility, yet we do it every day. When uncertain about the decision, get advice: ask another doctor, the pharmacist, or that nurse you know, and solicit opinions from a suitable online forum. But receive all this information critically and take responsibility for evaluating what it means to you.

How can I avoid hospitals?

This is the pivotal question, for it is not essential to turn over responsibility for wellness to someone else. The first and most important thing to do is change your attitude and realize that you, the individual, are in control. Then you can do things to increase your health, strengthen your immunity, and reduce your chances of ending up in a hospital.

Start by finding out about nutrition and supplementation. Initially, you may find that information about the large number of vitamins and minerals and how they act is confusing. Claims and counter-claims abound. However, you can find trustworthy websites and consider the advice provided. Such websites do not make claims to cure all cancers, prevent all diseases, or stop you aging so you can live forever. Government-sponsored websites are unlikely to be of help in keeping you healthy; typically, they will claim that nutritional supplements are unnecessary and potentially harmful. Consider all advice rather skeptically. Do not be swayed by academic qualifications. Many of the sites that provide the most reliable advice are authored by patients with a disease, who have become disillusioned by the inability of modern medicine to help.

Many people can improve their health and expected life span by simple actions. Smokers have a decision to make: they need to decide if their enjoyment of smoking outweighs the financial cost and the risks of heart disease, cancer, or other chronic illness. Added to this is the negative impact on their family. This is a personal choice. For some, the personal benefits of smoking trump the negative aspects. Some people, however, need to get help to overcome this addiction.

Dietary changes can greatly increase good health and longevity. Small modifications can have big effects; for example, lowering your intake of sucrose and high-fructose corn syrup. People who add sugar to their coffee or tea often think it tastes nicer and feel deprived without it. Remarkably, when a person stops taking sugar, their taste changes and, after a period, they find tea or coffee with sugar most unpalatable. Make the decision to drop the sugar and you will lose weight and have less risk of cancer and heart disease.

As a general rule, do not have health checks or tests unless you think there is a high chance you have the disease. As we have seen, such tests have high false-positive rates and may incorrectly indicate you have an illness. If this happens, you could risk the dangers of medication or even surgery when you are perfectly healthy. A doctor who wants you to have a test needs to explain why you should have it, the full risks of the test, and the accuracy (false-positive and false-negative rates, population incidence). If the doctor cannot provide this information, ask why not. Importantly, if you have a positive test result, ask for a retest, as it will provide at least some level of assurance that the first result was not an error.

Do not take any drugs for preventing a disease you do not have. Some doctors are suggesting polypills to prevent heart disease.[53] Such a pill might contain a combination of aspirin, three blood pressure–lowering drugs, and a statin drug to lower cholesterol. Healthy people taking a cocktail of multiple drugs are supposed to reduce their risk of heart disease, cancer, or whatever. In fact, a healthy person taking such medication can suffer side effects. The doctor will not know how the drugs will react together in the body over the long term. Importantly, the chance that a healthy person will benefit by taking multiple drugs to prevent a disease they do not have is remote. Polypharmacy will not make you healthier.

We know of no good evidence to support the use of statin drugs or aspirin for preventing heart disease in healthy people. Despite this, drugs to prevent illness are becoming popular with corporate medicine. The profits to be made by selling drugs to a large population of the healthy are immense. Moreover, it is a good way of making a profit from older drugs that are out of patent protection.

Before you take any drug, find out what it is for, determine why you need to take it, and check what benefit you can expect to get as an individual. If you do need the drug, find out the side effects, watch out for them, and make sure it is safe to take the drug for an extended period, if this is applicable.

Importantly, remember that for drugs proposed to prevent disease, often there is a safer nutritional supplement with a similar action or effect. Supplements typically have an array of health benefits and few, if any, side effects. Why take statins or aspirin to prevent heart disease when niacin, vitamin E, and fish oils are safe, effective, and cost less?

Start with a quality multivitamin and mineral tablet: make sure it is high dose and not one that provides only Recommended Dietary Allowance (RDA) levels. Check that it provides an adequate intake of vitamin D_3 (a minimum intake would be 2,000 IU each day and 5000 IU may give increased benefit). Add to that a natural, mixed vitamin E tablet (at least 600 IU each day) and vitamin C (start with low doses, such as 500 mg with each meal, and increase the dose gradually until you are consuming several grams a day). Each person is an individual with specific needs. As your knowledge of nutrition increases, decide which nutrients are the ones you need.

Begin with small changes to the diet, but don't be too hard on yourself. Changing eating habits is at least as difficult as stopping smoking, and just as important. If this were not the case, there would be far fewer obese people in the world. Take small steps in changing your diet and celebrate your achievements. You need to make positive changes that you can live with for the long term.

How can I take charge of my health care?

The first step in taking charge of your health care is to respect yourself. If you do not give yourself and your health suitable respect, do not imagine medical professionals will either. You need to expect to take the leading role in any decision making. Make sure your general practitioner is aware that you intend to be fully informed and to participate in your treatment decisions.

Find a Doctor Who Will Support You

Nowadays, doctors are being encouraged to support participative medicine. For example, the website of the U.K. General Medical Council (GMC), the body that regulates and registers doctors in the United Kingdom, advises doctors to approach patients in the following way:

Relationships based on openness, trust, and good communication will enable you to work in partnership with your patients to address their individual needs. To fulfill your role in the doctor-patient partnership, the doctor must:

- Be polite, considerate, and honest

- Treat patients with dignity

- Treat each patient as an individual

- Respect patients' privacy and right to confidentiality

- Support patients in caring for themselves to improve and maintain their health

- Encourage patients who have knowledge about their condition to use this when they are making decisions about their care

In its description of the duties of a doctor, the GMC encourages a participative approach as follows:

- Patients must be able to trust doctors with their lives and health. To justify that trust, you must show respect for human life and you must:
  - Work in partnership with patients
  - Listen to patients and respond to their concerns and preferences
  - Give patients the information they want or need in a way they can understand
  - Respect patients' right to reach decisions with you about their treatment and care

If your doctor adheres to these or similar guidelines, you can hope to have found a helpful ally in avoiding hospitals and maintaining your health.

If you have a psychiatric problem or are in danger from dementia, ensure that you have intelligent friends or relatives to take care of your health and well-being. Be sure to choose advocates who will put your needs first and not be cowed by medical authority.

You need a diagnosis when you get sick. If possible, Google your symptoms before you see your doctor. When the doctor provides a diagnosis, check the verdict against the symptoms yourself. Try to find out if any other diseases fit the symptoms. If you do not agree with the diagnosis, tell the doctor and, if necessary, get a second opinion. If you do agree, find out about the possible treatments. Check the websites that specialize in your disease. When the doctor suggests a treatment, ask why that approach is likely to be the best. Expect an answer based on a rational assessment of the evidence.

What if we do it ourselves and do it wrong?

Much of the fear of doing something wrong vanishes as we become more knowledgeable. There is no fence around health information that prevents us from learning it. Likewise, there is no law preventing us from using our acquired knowledge to benefit our health. The key is to gain the knowledge by wanting to learn and by wanting the responsibility for our own well-being. Your aim is to reduce your risk of harm and ensure the appropriate treatment. Naturally, you cannot achieve zero risk. Patients thinking for themselves and taking responsibility means health costs will be far lower and malpractice lawyers will lose business.

Taking responsibility does not mean going against medical advice. It means working with the advice, wisdom, and knowledge of your physician. Expecting your doctor to treat you like an intelligent human being, on something like equal terms, is reasonable. The doctor is there to help prevent you from making a mistake.

Participative medicine also helps the doctor. If you participate and take some of the responsibility for a decision, it is far less likely that the physician will be blamed for any errors. You are checking the symptoms against the diagnosis, the treatment against the disease, and avoiding drug side effects. Participative medicine has an objective—to avoid the side effects and mistakes that are a plague in modern medicine. You and your doctor have the same aim, for you to be healthy and not be harmed by medicine.

Don't doctors and hospitals today have open minds?

Some doctors are embracing participative medicine, but others may resist what they see as a challenge to their position and standing. A general practitioner with an open mind will listen to patients and their wishes. If your doctor is resistant to participative medicine, use of supplements, or nutritional approaches, find another physician.

Medical doctors go to medical schools, where they learn to practice medicine. Most medical personnel are unfamiliar with nutritional treatments. Many disregard nutritional supplementation and preventive health care, without knowing what they are dismissing. This is a great loss to the doctor as well as to the public.

The new medicine may, ultimately, be based on good nutrition and prevention, leaving our current health-care treatments as a minor final option. This ideal depends on intelligent patients becoming involved and making choices to maintain their own standard of health.

Mainstream medicine is not going to concur with your ideas, is it?

Probably not. This book is about the failings of corporate medicine and how patients can avoid doctor-induced illness. We would be surprised if some doctors did not consider the book suitable for burning. The figures on adverse events in hospitals are devastating; something needs to be done.

Many doctors will agree that medicine needs improving. Our suggestion is to build on recent initiatives, such as participative medicine. We simply want medicine to become more rational. We think a person has a right to reduce the risks incurred in modern medicine. People can check and make sure they are not taking unnecessary risks. This is a rational response by patients.

Can natural healing really beat serious illness?

Natural therapies are not just another way to fight disease—the aim is to prevent the illness in the first place. Natural healing modifies the basics, such as diet and lifestyle, which are the major determinants of illness today. They are also habits that are difficult to change; no one is following you around checking that you eat right, take exercise, and live happily.

A distinguishing feature of most natural therapies is that they are straightforward enough to do safely on your own at home. Drugs and surgery are not inherently safe. With drugs, a chemical or poison is added to the body. In surgery, an organ or part of the body is cut, mutilated, or removed.

Treatment is needed when a person has a chronic disease or becomes ill. In such cases, we suggest the first approach should be using diet and supplements to obtain benefit without harm. This should be done with the knowledge and advice of a physician. In many cases, disease can be cured or effectively treated by nutritional supplementation alone.

Why do people have more confidence in hospitals than nutrition?

Most of the devastating impact of hospital failures is hidden. Confidence in corporate medicine is, however, changing. Over half of Americans will see an alternative practitioner this year. More people are aware that hospital-derived infections are becoming endemic and widespread. People need to realize that there is no direct evidence that modern medicine, taken as a whole, is helpful. It may harm more than it helps.

If nutritional medicine is effective, why don't doctors use it?

It is not rational to expect corporate medicine to tell you how to avoid their services by using alternatives. Hospitals, doctors, and pharmaceutical companies share a common Achilles' heel—they all profit from disease. Follow the money and you will understand that it is not in their interest to support the competition.

However, the majority of doctors are ethical. A recent study found that doctors and nurses were as likely as members of the general public to take vitamins. The Health-care Professionals Impact Study in 2009 found that 72 percent of physicians and 89 percent of nurses used dietary supplements.[54] Over half of doctors (51 percent) and nurses (59 percent) used supplements regularly, and many took supplements for overall health and wellness. Both doctors and nurses recommended supplements to their patients. Medicine is changing its head-in-the-sand attitude. If your doctor tells you that supplements do not work, we suggest you realize that he or she is in the minority.

What is the legality of all this?

Participating in your treatment is not illegal—it is good medicine. We are not suggesting you step outside the law or have dangerous treatments. Rather, we are proposing that patients act rationally and become actively involved in their own care.

Self-care means accepting some risk and much responsibility. You accept that your doctors are human and can make mistakes. There is an implicit agreement: your doctor respects your involvement and you accept that errors can occur. As a participator in medical decisions, you are much less likely to take legal action against the hospital unless they make an outlandish mistake. If you are not prepared to accept this level of responsibility, then participative medicine may not be for you.

MOVE TOWARD SELF-RELIANCE

We will get health care for individuals when they take responsibility for their own health. People need specific instruction on how exactly to do this, and they have not been getting it. This book is expressly designed to both educate and motivate the general reader toward self-reliance. Our main aim is for readers to become more rational patients, with the confidence to think for themselves.

CHAPTER 8

The Power of Nutrition

*"The effect of this state of things is to make the medical
profession a conspiracy to hide its own shortcomings.
No doubt the same may be said of all professions.
They are all conspiracies against the laity."*
—George Bernard Shaw (1856–1950)

The relationship between nutrition and health has a long history. There is little excuse for the failure of hospitals to provide adequate nutrition. Suitable nutrition, provision of rest, warmth, cleanliness, and other care are paramount in the treatment of ill health. Supplements are preferable to drugs partly because, being natural constituents of the diet, there is less risk of side effects. Fortunately, many individuals have taken responsibility for their own health and are supplementing their diet with additional vitamins and minerals.[1]

One example mentioned earlier is the use of vitamin B_3 (niacin) to lower cholesterol. Recently, niacin was shown to be more effective than a cholesterol-lowering drug, Zetia (ezetimibe).[2] Zetia inhibits absorption of cholesterol from the gut. However, cholesterol in the diet does not contribute much to blood levels. The body makes cholesterol in the liver, so if you get more in the diet, the liver makes correspondingly less. Conversely, if less is provided by the diet, the liver manufactures more. It is therefore unsurprising that Zetia should largely fail at lowering cholesterol in the blood. Slow-release niacin appears to be more protective against cardiovascular disease and is less expensive. Niacin has been used in this way for over fifty years and provided "the most potent therapy" for altering blood cholesterol.

When the media report the benefits of a supplement, they typically add some condition as to why it should not be used. In this case, news reports stated that the (slow-release) niacin used was a special prescription-only form not available in health food stores.[3] We hope these statements were made in ignorance of the availability of niacin and other B vitamins as over-the-counter supplements. Misinformation about health is ubiquitous in the media and many medical journals consistently bias their conclusions against nutrition and health. Suggesting that slow-release niacin is not available as a supplement is a minor example.

In fact, niacin is widely available in both standard and slow-release forms. About 9 million Americans take the rather expensive and useless Zetia, whereas less than 3 million take the more effective and less costly niacin supplements. The drug has a long list of side effects, including headache, fatigue, gastrointestinal upset, hypersensitivity reactions, anaphylaxis, hepatitis, and so on.[4] In contrast, the main side effect of taking sufficient B vitamins is excellent good health. Dr. Hoffer would inform his patients that the main side effect from niacin is that they would live longer. And then he would wryly add, "Is that a problem for you?"

ANTIOXIDANT MISINFORMATION

Antioxidants are one of the main targets for media misinformation. An antioxidant delivers electrons to the body's cells. Indeed, our bodies burn food partly to supply energy but also to generate antioxidant electrons. Without antioxidants, we might age rapidly like butter going rancid on a hot day. Antioxidants are essential to life, health, and well-being. However, the potential of antioxidants to prevent disease means potential competition to the use of drugs and an implicit pressure on corporate medicine.

One role of antioxidants is to prevent cancer. The medical literature abounds with reports and reviews that both support and contradict the idea that antioxidants are beneficial. Many of the reports are poorly designed studies, especially those that purport to show antioxidants have little or no benefit. One review of antioxidant supplements found little evidence that the antioxidants prevent gastrointestinal cancers.[5] The implicit claims of the paper were simply wrong. First, there are numerous antioxidants in the diet, which were not covered by the review. Any one of these antioxidants might be effective. Despite this, the authors implied that their results apply to all dietary antioxidant supplements. The authors, editors, and reviewers of this paper were surely aware that the broad claims of this paper were misleading. It concluded that, alone or in combination, antioxidants "do not seem to have much effect." Not seeming to have much effect is an unusually vague set of words to find in a scientific paper. The authors were covering their claims carefully.

The reviewers were right to have hedged their bets, since claims for the beneficial effects of antioxidants have often used far larger doses than those covered in their paper. It may even be that, in biochemical terms, they were not studying antioxidants at all. For example, the review covered intakes of vitamin E from only 30 to 600 IU each day. However, to provide antioxidant benefit requires much higher doses, taken for a prolonged period. An intake of 1,600 IU a day will have an antioxidant effect, if taken for many weeks.[6] Even an intake of 3,200 IU will require about sixteen weeks to generate a maximum antioxidant effect. Furthermore, beneficial claims specify the natural form of vitamin E, not the synthetic form, but this was not made clear in the review. Importantly, "vitamin E" does not exist as a single molecule: there are multiple forms, including eight main naturally occurring types (four tocopherols and four tocotrienols).

In this same review, selenium and beta-carotene were also studied. The element selenium also occurs in many different forms, both naturally and in supplements. Like many substances, selenium can act either as an oxidant or an antioxidant, depending on the form, the conditions, and the dose. Beta carotene is similarly Janus-faced and can act either as an oxidant or an antioxidant. The authors of the study describe these substances simply as antioxidants, apparently not realizing their true nature.

According to these authors, beta carotene appears to increase morbidity. However, this finding was based on two dominating large studies, involving men who were heavy smokers and some who had been exposed to asbestos. A third study, on non-smoking physicians, did not show any toxic effect from beta carotene. These results might be predicted from the antioxidant action of beta carotene. Throughout their bodies, smokers have a massive oxidant pressure as a result of the smoke they inhale. In such conditions, antioxidants of the beta carotene type can act as oxidants, unless they are supported by a second source of antioxidants, such as massive intakes of vitamin C. Antioxidant supplements work together synergistically.

The effect magnitudes of the low doses of antioxidants were probably below the sensitivity of the trials. The authors are, in effect, reporting the effects of minor biases in the experimental design or procedure. In studies of "antioxidants" and lung cancer, similar small increases in risk are reported with beta carotene in some studies,[7] but not in all.[8] Most so-called gold-standard studies of this type are known to be wrong![9] This form of trial, with this intake of nutrients, can be repeated indefinitely, with varying results. Sometimes, beta carotene will seem to cause cancer, and other times it apparently prevents cancer. Such are the benefits of so-called evidence-based medicine. People are becoming aware of the contradictory results of these trials, which are likely to do little more than bring medical science into disrepute.

It is important to know the exact methods used in this study. The study used a large population of male smokers, aged 50–69. One group was given a synthetic form of vitamin E (dl-alpha tocopherol). Another group was given 20 mg of beta carotene, which is a low dose. A third group was on placebo, and the fourth group received both antioxidants.

We have some observations on this methodology. In lungs ravaged by oxidants from tobacco smoke, the antioxidant potential of the beta carotene would be overwhelmed. We have explained how low doses of vitamin E will not act as antioxidants. In this case, the synthetic (dl) form was used, despite the widely known fact that claims for benefit reside in the particular molecular forms (d) of the natural vitamin. Testing of synthetic supplements does not address the health claims for the natural supplements. If someone asked us to design a misleading study to apparently demonstrate that antioxidant supplements were ineffective or harmful, we might use a similar approach, molecules, and doses to the ones in these particular studies. Experiments can be set up to fail.

Having dealt with the main elements of this flawed trial, we find multiple related issues. Contrary to popular belief, large-scale trials are often subject to biases, which can subtly alter the results. Small differences found in large studies, as in this case, should be considered highly suspect. The subjects smoked five or more cigarettes daily for over thirty-five years. They were followed in the study for five to eight years. But the beta carotene group had smoked on average for one year more than the control group, thus the groups were not comparable. In the control group, the men with the highest blood levels of these two antioxidants showed the lowest incidence of lung cancer. The dl-alpha tocopherol (synthetic vitamin E) group showed a small reduction in the incidence of lung cancer, but this was not statistically significant.

In the beta carotene group, an 18 percent increase in incidence of the cancer was claimed. However, note the use of relative statistics, which amplify the result and increase its apparent importance. Of 14,560 men on beta carotene, 474 developed cancer, while out of 14,573 men not on beta carotene, 402 did. The actual incidence increased from 2.76 percent for the control group to 3.26 percent for the treated group. This minor difference (0.5 percent) is of little clinical importance and could reflect a minor bias in the experimental setup, even though it is statistically significant because of the large number of participants in the study. Expressed in plain language, the incidence in each group was about three per 100. However, dividing 3.26 by 2.76 gives 1.18, or an 18 percent increase. This much larger number is stressed and may be the only figure an unwary reader will remember. With large sample sizes such as these, a minor variation can be artificially inflated into a major finding.

There was something odd about the Finnish group of men in the study. The authors reported that one in three of the men on beta carotene developed yellow skin. This is totally foreign to our experience. For example, Dr. Hoffer has started at least 500 subjects on this amount of beta carotene (and far more), yet he never encountered yellowing of the skin with anything close to this low dose. It does occur, but with far higher doses. This observation could suggest that the liver function of these heavy smokers was compromised and they were unable to deal with normal doses of beta carotene.

Cancer is often present and undetectable in patients long before it is finally discovered. A preventive study should start before any tumors are in progress, which could mean many years. With this group of heavy smokers, it is likely that a large fraction had already started developing cancer. It was therefore a mixed study, consisting of treatment for those already with cancer, and prevention for those who were initially free of the disease. Treatment and prevention of cancer with antioxidant supplements require different dose levels and have different mechanisms of action.

These large studies are an expensive waste of resources that could be more usefully employed. The results demonstrate nothing of use but are potentially misleading. If you supplement with tiny doses of synthetic vitamin E, nothing much will happen. If you give heavy chronic smokers 20 mg

Tricking Patients?

The *Courier Mail*, an Australian newspaper, reported a possible cancer cure.[11] Ecobiotics, a Queensland company, claimed an extract of blushwood fruit could kill cancer cells. Blushwood is found in native rainforests. The extract, called EBC-46, was described by Dr. Victoria Gordon as "proving to be something exceptional" and "the tumor literally liquefies." The extract is easy to administer and appears to be safe with few side effects. It was said to work on several different forms of cancer, including melanoma and bone tumors. It may also work on breast, colon, and prostate cancers.

Blushwood extract was tried in fifty dogs, as well as cats and horses.[12] Tumors were said to disintegrate within twenty-four hours, and healing was rapid. Elton Buchanan, from Melbourne, was the owner of a Great Dane that was treated for an inoperable nasal tumor. When excited, the dog would rasp and snuffle and have a nosebleed. One treatment with EBC-46 produced a rapid therapeutic response and, three months later, the symptoms disappeared completely.

We are not particularly locked onto the reported cancer-killing properties of this herbal extract; there are numerous safe cancer-killing substances with similar properties.[13] Unfortunately, the sick are actively discouraged from benefiting from safe therapies by the active restriction of patient choice. In this case, Dr. Gordon, CEO of Ecobiotics, was reported as explaining that it was "immoral, illegal, and unscientific" for patients to demand the extract before it was officially approved. She did not "want to kill the enthusiasm of all the wonderful research, but until it is proven it will do the job, we recommend they go with proven and conventional treatments."

We do not wish to criticize Dr. Gordon and we wish her success with her project. Her research initiative may be original, but she is responding to the media in a standard way. Doctors and scientists reporting research on nutrients and herbs appear to be required by corporate medicine to always provide a warning not to take the supplement. So, for example, if your clinical trial shows that high intakes of vitamin E prevent heart disease, you are expected to say "but don't take supplements, at least not yet" and provide a reason, such as further research is required or there may be unknown safety issues. Dr. Gordon was merely being conventional.

However, such conventional concern for cancer patients is irrational and may cause them great harm. In this case, the Therapeutic Goods Administration would take up to seven years to authorize the use of EBC-46. So, a terminal patient would need to wait until after they had died to try the treatment.

The rational patient's approach is to say that EBC-46 is an option for their terminal cancer. A dying cancer patient has a right to make their own decision about treatment. In this case, the treatment appears to be safe. It may cause harm in humans, but there is no evidence for this suggestion. A patient having the treatment has a chance of surviving the cancer or, at least, of living longer in good health. There would appear to be a good chance that they could achieve large benefit; it might save their life. There is a risk of harm, but this currently appears to be small for the individual patient. A rational patient with terminal cancer might choose to try the treatment.

At the time of writing, people can apply to get blushwood treatment for their dog, in a clinical trial, but are discouraged in attempting to save their own lives. Given that a patient's rational choice might be to try the treatment, we see no justification for the idea that it would be immoral. It is not wicked or depraved to make a decision to try to save your life, with no harm to others. It is most certainly not unscientific to engage in a rational treatment decision. Moreover, EBC-46 is not a controlled drug. Rational choice is not "immoral, illegal, and unscientific."

These reports for blushwood extract killing cancer are unremarkable: selectively killing cancer cells, without harming the host, appears to be surprisingly easy. It is not a breakthrough, as there are numerous substances, including vitamin C, that can safely kill cancer cells. The difficulty is in working out how to use such substances to maximum benefit, a process that is discouraged and prevented by corporate medicine.

Patients are often tricked out of making decisions about their own health care by well-meaning but irrational platitudes. Do not be a victim of corporate medicine. There is no such thing as a "scientifically proven" treatment, as science abhors certainty and proof. Patients should consider the evidence for so-called unproven therapies and think for themselves. It may save a life—your life.

of beta carotene, their incidence of lung cancer may or may not change. The authors do point out that "findings regarded as showing supplementation to be beneficial or harmful may occur by chance." Presumably, they had a suspicion that they were merely reporting experimental bias.

Beta carotene is converted in the body to vitamin A. The protective effect of dietary vitamin A against lung cancer was reported in 1975.[10] Since then, a large number of studies have indicated that higher levels of vitamin A in food are associated with decreased incidence of cancer. Laboratory experiments and animal studies have also found that the vitamin is protective against cancer. The general rule is to treat epidemiology and large-scale trials as suspect. The evidence that such social studies provide is often ambivalent and misleading.

DIET IS NOT ENOUGH

Doctors often answer patients' requests for information on supplementation by asserting that, if people consume fruits and vegetables, they will get all the vitamins they need from food. In reality, that cannot be known. It is only an idea at best and a legend at worst. Data on nutrients and health is far too limited. Doctors assume that they are being scientific when they make these claims, without realizing it is simply historical prejudice.

Following the discovery of vitamins, it was found that the acute deficiency diseases did not occur provided a person had a small intake of the required vitamin. In other words, if you consume a few milligrams of vitamin C, you will not suffer the horrors of acute scurvy (teeth falling out, rotten gums, joint pains, bruising, death). As a result, doctors assumed that only small intakes of the vitamins were necessary. This idea was even incorporated into the definition of a vitamin, as a substance that, in minute quantities, is essential to normal metabolism.

However, *just because a minute quantity of a vitamin will prevent acute deficiency disease does not mean that it is the optimal dose.* In the long term, for example, low intakes could lead to chronic illnesses. This hypothesis has been repeatedly suggested over the last fifty years for a number of vitamins but has not been tested. It is not scientific for doctors to say that we need only small intakes of vitamins, as there is not enough evidence to support such claims. The assertion that supplements are unnecessary is a statement of ignorance rather than scientific enlightenment.

Shortage of vitamins and other nutrients may result in chronic disease, including heart attacks, strokes, many cancers, arthritis, dementia, psychosis, and so on. There are no studies to show that this is not the case. Nor is it easy to see how a scientific study could be conducted within a reasonable period. If, for example, dementia was a result of long-term shortage of vitamin B_{12}, it would require a study extending over many decades to demonstrate the effect. Such trials are not performed.

Many people live on junk food and do not even reach the low Recommended Dietary Allowance (RDA) levels of vitamin intake. Even in First World countries, hunger and malnutrition are still with us. The authorities and the media would like us to believe that, in our affluent countries,

The Vitamin C Man

Biochemist Irwin Stone introduced Linus Pauling to vitamin C. Dr. Pauling remembered this highly influential first contact, when Dr. Stone sent him some papers on vitamin C that he had just published. "The 3,000 milligrams per day that he recommended is 50 times the RDA," said Dr. Pauling. "My wife and I began taking this amount of the vitamin . . . (and) the severe colds that I had suffered from several times a year all of my life no longer occurred. After a few years, I increased my intake of vitamin C to 100 times, then 200 times, and then 300 times the RDA (now 18,000 mg per day)."[18]

Nearly fifty years ago, Dr. Stone postulated that humans have inherited a genetic trait to need but not manufacture ascorbic acid (vitamin C). This innate dependency may be made up for in diet, but not easily. The government's Recommended Dietary Allowance (RDA) for vitamin C is far less than the amount produced daily by most other mammals.

Dr. Stone's 1972 book, *The Healing Factor: Vitamin C Against Disease*, contains a description of the decades he spent researching the substance.[19] It summarized the apparently successful vitamin C treatment of infections (bacterial and viral), allergies, asthma, poisoning, ulcers, and eye diseases including glaucoma. The potential role of vitamin C in treating cancer, heart disease, diabetes, fractures, bladder and kidney diseases, tetanus, shock, wounds, and pregnancy complications was also described. Despite the claims of great benefit, none of this work seems to be of interest to modern medicine.

children are well fed and educated, but even in the United States, hungry children are an increasing problem.[14] The consequences are often more invidious than realized. Poor children are more likely to display behavioral problems and end up on antipsychotic medication.[15] This medication is typically prescribed by a nonspecialist doctor, rather than a psychiatrist. Such problems have been predicted to result from nutritional deficiencies.[16] Doctors are doping children into submission rather than helping to provide adequate nutrition. Low-cost vitamin and mineral supplements would ameliorate many of the harmful effects of childhood malnutrition. People are short of nutrients and many do not realize the harm it is doing to themselves and their children.

Every so often, a leading researcher rediscovers the benefits of supplementation. Dr. Irwin Stone famously introduced Linus Pauling to vitamin C, and Dr. Hoffer did the same with niacin. These events led to the foundation of orthomolecular medicine as a discipline. Dr. Roger Williams described how we are all unique individuals with particular nutritional needs. More recently, Dr. Bruce Ames found that low levels of nutrients cause multiple DNA mutations and increase the risk of cancer.[17] Unfortunately, corporate medicine ignores these findings, preferring to maintain the profitable status quo.

STATINS ARE NOT NUTRITIOUS

Corporate medicine's rejection of nutritional therapy can appear obsessive. A recent study suggested that statins might be used to help prevent diseases that are likely to be due to nutritional deficiency. Writing in the *New England Journal of Medicine,* the JUPITER study group described a study in which statin drugs were apparently successful in preventing heart disease and stroke.[20] The aim was to find out whether statin drugs could provide any benefit to people with low cholesterol. This was not a purely academic question. Cholesterol-lowering drugs are normally used for people with high cholesterol. If it could be shown that they could also help people with low cholesterol, it would mean a larger market and increased sales for the drug company.

Heart disease and stroke are caused by inflammation in the arterial wall. High C-reactive protein levels in the blood are associated with inflammation and thus are linked with heart disease or stroke. The subjects in this trial had low cholesterol and elevated inflammation (C-reactive protein).

The authors concluded that, in apparently healthy persons with elevated C-reactive protein levels, rosuvastatin (Crestor) significantly reduced the incidence of major cardiovascular events.

Since this was a profitable statin drug, the study received widespread publicity. Its claim, that the statin lowers the risk of heart attack by approximately one half, is technically correct though highly misleading. The reported annual incidence of coronary events was 37 people in 10,000 (controls) and 17 people in 10,000 (treated); similar results were reported for risk of stroke. When expressed as a proportion, a 46 percent improvement (17/37) sounds large. In absolute terms, however, an improvement of 20 events (37 – 17) in 10,000 people known to be at risk sounds less impressive: the already slight risk was reduced by just one event for every 500 people treated!

The widespread publicity following the release of this study suggested that millions of healthy people could cut their risk of heart disease by taking statins.[21] Reporters also claimed that statins could cut the risk of heart attack for "everyone."[22] This was inaccurate and incorrect. The study did not include normal healthy people, only a sample of a relatively small number of people who were suffering from inflammation (increased C-reactive protein), a known cause of heart disease and stroke. Out of 89,890 people considered for inclusion, only 17,802 people (19.8 percent) met the specific criteria of poor health for the study. Widespread prescription of statins to healthy people is not supported by these findings.

A rational doctor would not consider prescribing this drug for a patient based on these results. The statin drug might perhaps produce a minor reduction in risk in the population, at a high financial cost. This risk in a population cannot be directly applied to a single individual. But if we assume that the risk could be applied, an individual patient would pay $1,000 a year to lower their risk of a heart attack or a stroke by one chance in 500. That is a large fee for a small return, even before we consider the risk of statin side effects.

People who understand nutrition and inflammation consider statins a sucker's bet. The fact that statins produce a modest improvement is unsurprising, since they are known to lower inflammation, as do many nutritional supplements. As health writer Bill Sardi has pointed out, Crestor lowers C-reactive protein by 37 percent, but vitamin E lowers it by 32 percent,[23] and vitamin C by 25.3 percent.[24] These effects are similar to those of statins and would be expected to provide comparable benefits, without side effects and at a much lower cost.

Crestor and other statin drugs have serious side effects. The incidence of established side-effects, such as rhabdomyolysis (0.3 per 10,000 per year), myopathy (1.1 per 10,000), and peripheral neuropathy (1.2 per 10,000 per year) seems low,[25] but may be underestimated, as it takes time to establish long-term side effects. These preliminary figures imply that for ten people who avoid a cardiovascular event, at least one previously healthy person will suffer a non-trivial side effect of the statin drug.

The JUPITER group who carried out this study reported a statistically significant increase in diabetes in the statin group, compared to the placebo group. Over the course of the study, this corresponds to an increased risk of approximately 61 in 10,000 people. In fact, the number of extra people on statins who were reported to have become diabetic was greater than the number who avoided a heart attack! In the long term, these people might have shorter lives and be at greater risk of heart disease. Notably, the JUPITER study was stopped early, which even the authors admit prevents assessment of how side effects might outweigh reported benefits in the longer term. The study was intended to last three to five years and criteria for stopping were not included in the original published design.[26]

JUPITER stands for "Justification for the Use of Statins in Prevention: an Intervention Trial Evaluating Rosuvastatin." The reader might well think this "justification" sounds more like a marketing plan than a scientific endeavor. The researchers did not address the underlying cause of the inflammation and increased C-reactive protein; they simply treated the condition with drugs. In many cases, raised C-reactive protein is a result of nutritional deficiency.[27] Several nutritional supplements inhibit inflammation and lower C-reactive protein, without causing known side effects. Deficiencies in vitamins A,[28] B$_6$, C, E, folate, carotenoids, lycopene,[29] and selenium are associated with raised C-reactive protein.[30] People at risk could supplement their diet and restore their health, without using expensive drugs to conceal their underlying sickness.

THE GOLDEN ERA IS OVER

Back in the 1930s, headline news about vitamins was surprisingly honest. This was the golden era of vitamin discovery: Nobel prizes were given to pioneers who discovered, identified, or isolated them. There are some exceptions, such as Dr. Roger Williams, who discovered pantothenic acid (vitamin B_5) yet did not become a Nobel laureate, though he received many other honors. Announcements in the science of nutrition were typically followed with great interest, and people realized that vitamins would prevent otherwise incurable diseases. Studies using the newly identified vitamins were carried out as soon as they became available. An example of this was Dr. William Kaufman's use of niacinamide (a form of niacin) to treat joint dysfunction in the 1930s, only a few years after niacin was identified. Some of the most successful nutritional studies were conducted by curious scientists in those early years. These reports gradually tailed off with the introduction of the antibiotics and the steroid "wonder drugs."

Medicine seems to have gone from one extreme to the other. Studies only a few years old may be ignored. For hundreds, if not thousands, of years, physicians followed the ideas of the ancients, from the mythical Asklepios to Hippocrates and Galen. Nowadays, however, they often assume that anything old must be inferior to the new. Neither method is sensible. *Evidence should be considered on its merits, not its age.*

The pioneering physicians who laid the foundations of modern medicine were not handicapped by the requirement to perform double-blind, randomized clinical trials. They had little funding for their studies, so these early scientists had to think and design good experiments. But now, such clinical or "anecdotal" studies are condemned and considered largely useless. They do not meet a set of statistical standards for social medicine, described as "evidence based," introduced since the 1970s. We prefer well-designed experiments to statistics. In the words of Ernest Rutherford, the great experimental physicist, "If your experiment needs statistics, you ought to have done a better experiment."

Unfortunately, the main purpose of the modern double-blind, controlled trial appears to be persuading regulating bodies that a product of corporate medicine should be released onto the unsuspecting public. Organizations without the resources of the major drug companies are unable to meet the regulatory standards. A secondary consideration is marketing. As we have seen, a large-scale trial can be used to amplify the minor effects of a drug and persuade doctors and patients that it is some kind of breakthrough. Clinical trials have become so large they have created a de facto monopoly. Epidemiology and large clinical trials are turning medicine into social science. Dr. Rutherford's view of social science is also most apt: "The only possible conclusion the social sciences can draw is: some do, some don't." This agrees with modern interpretations that most clinical trials are simply wrong.[31] Unfortunately, a good deal of harm may be done before a typical drug is found wanting and the side effects discovered.

Small-scale studies, using targeted subjects and designed to look for major differences between the treated and the control group, are much more likely to be of value than are huge and expensive trials. The vitamin pioneers used the vitamin-as-prevention paradigm, which played a useful role in discovering and isolating essential nutrients. The initial idea was that vitamin supplements should only be used where the person is deficient in those nutrients. This seemed obvious: there would be no point giving extra vitamin C if people are already getting all that they need. It therefore became important to determine whether populations really did need extra supplements and then only to provide those in short supply. Unfortunately, it is extremely difficult to determine the requirements necessary to prevent chronic disease, such as atherosclerosis and cancer. It was hoped that small intakes would suffice for good health. This assumption has potentially caused millions to suffer debilitating disease and early death.

The truth is, it is not known whether people are woefully deficient in nutrients, such as vitamin C. However, there is strong suggestive evidence that many chronic diseases and conditions associated with aging are primarily the result of long-term nutritional deficiency.

SUPPLEMENTS TO TAKE
BEFORE GOING TO THE HOSPITAL

Asking for guidance on nutrition from a doctor is a bit like trying to buy a new Honda from a Ford dealer. You may be told "Just eat a balanced diet" or "Supplements are unnecessary." A major reason that hospitals are so dangerous is because corporate medicine downgrades the importance of nutrition. It is irrational to ask the people who are responsible for a problem to provide the solution.

Nutritionists, dietitians, and physicians often maintain that vitamin deficiencies are rare in our modern civilization. For example, the U.S. Food and Drug Administration (FDA) has removed the need for B-vitamin information from food nutrition labels because they perceive it to be unnecessary. Nevertheless, nutritional supplements are essential for preventing illness. Only about one in ten Americans consumes sufficient nutrients in their diet.[32] In 1990, it was reported that 45 percent of Americans did not take fruit or juice daily, and 22 percent consumed no servings of a vegetable.[33] Only 27 percent ate three or more helpings of vegetables and 29 percent took two or more servings of fruit, as then recommended by the U.S. Departments of Agriculture and of Health and Human Services. No wonder we have so many hospitals.

Vitamin A

Studies confirm that vitamin A deficiency weakens immune function, thus we all require an adequate provision of this vitamin. Beta carotene is the precursor of vitamin A, so a safe way to obtain this vitamin is to take beta carotene, which the body will convert into vitamin A as needed. This method also avoids the risk of overdose, especially during pregnancy. Vitamin A is one of the few vitamins that produces significant toxicity if taken in excess. Excessively large doses of preformed vitamin A can depress immune function, but beta carotene does not appear to have this negative effect.

Beta carotene supplements strengthen the immune system by helping the body to build more helper T cells.[34] Ideally, the body can derive about 10,000 IU of vitamin A activity from each 6 milligrams of beta carotene consumed. The actual conversion is likely to be less than this figure, however. Small amounts of beta carotene (20 mg or so) are likely to show no benefit, even though the predicted yield would be over 30,000 IU of vitamin A activity.

Following surgery, the white blood cell count usually decreases. Vitamin A acts as an immune stimulant and prevents this postoperative problem.[35] We suggest beta carotene supplementation should be taken alongside dynamic flow intakes of vitamin C.[36] This requires at least 500 mg of vitamin C to be taken several times a day (every four to six hours). The maximum intake is limited by bowel tolerance and produces loose stool. The dose of vitamin C should be gradually increased to just below the maximum tolerable.

B Vitamins

Deficiency of B vitamins can be devastating. The disease beri-beri means

"I cannot, I cannot," relating to severe weakness and exhaustion. This previously incurable condition was found to be a deficiency of vitamin B_1 (thiamine). Eating whole brown rice instead of polished white rice was enough to effect a remarkable cure from the fatigue that had resisted drug therapy. A similar weakness and lassitude is found with deficiency of vitamin B_3 (niacin).[37]

In the body, food is broken down into simple molecules such as glucose, a sugar and the cells' main source of immediate energy. A major part of the complex process that converts glucose to energy is called the Krebs, or citric acid, cycle. Without the B-complex vitamins, this elaborate energy-releasing biochemical pathway grinds to a halt. The four B-vitamins most involved with the cellular energy cycle are thiamine, niacin, pantothenic acid and riboflavin. We have focused on the first two, as the last two are reasonably well provided, even in modern diets: riboflavin (B_2) is in all milk products; pantothenic acid is found in most cells, so it cannot easily be avoided in food.

Scientific research indicates that vitamin B deficiencies weaken immunity.[38] We suggest a high quality "B-50" supplement should be taken *twice* each day. In addition to those mentioned above, this should provide B_6, B_{12}, folic acid, and biotin.

Vitamin C

Vitamin C can improve your chances of surviving a hospital stay. Massive doses of vitamin C have been described as successfully boosting the immune system for fifty years. Back in the 1940s, Dr. Frederick Klenner pioneered vitamin C therapeutics, giving exceptionally large intakes for a wide variety of viral illnesses.[39] For over half a century, a stream of doctors has observed and confirmed the benefits of vitamin C in shock and illness.[40]

Notably, Dr. Robert Cathcart has published his successes with enormous doses of vitamin C for many viral illnesses. Even among patients with fully developed AIDS, improved length of life and quality of life are the rule, not the exception.[41] In 1988, Dr. Ian Brighthope published his book *The AIDS Fighters,* describing how massive doses of vitamin C restored patients in the terminal stages of AIDS.[42] However, his observations were ignored. Some AIDS patients took up the therapy, but many did not appreciate the magnitude of the doses needed. The increased energy

A Surgeon Converted by Vitamin C

Robert Cathcart (1932–2007) was a doctor who based his work on basic science as well as his direct experience and observation of patients. His surgical training was at Stanford Hospital and he was an instructor of orthopedic surgery at Stanford from 1966 to 1967. His first major contribution was to design a hip prosthesis used in over 100,000 hip replacements. However, he abandoned surgery and corporate medicine when he observed the power of large intakes of vitamin C. First, he tried treating himself for a persistent allergy. Later, he was amazed at the response of his patients. Dr. Cathcart used far greater doses of vitamin C than popularly imagined—he reported the effects of intakes up to 300 grams a day. More recently, Dr. Cathcart became well known for his work on the concept of bowel tolerance as a way of finding the amount of vitamin C a person needs.

Dr. Cathcart reported his observations of immediate and unparalleled recovery in a range of illnesses, from the common cold to AIDS. Unsurprisingly, his reports were ignored. In his own words: "In 1978, a NBC reporter who had just won the Peabody (the rattlesnake in the mailbox story) did a piece on my work. She had two photographers who were shooting film on several of my patients who had been cured suddenly of several infectious diseases (especially on the treatment of hepatitis) with intravenous vitamin C and massive doses of ascorbic acid orally. She said this was the best story she had ever done. But the story was squelched the day it was to be aired. I wonder if they still have that story in the can in their library."

Dr. Cathcart's work was based on rational observation in patients. He said that other doctors never accused him of lying—they just thought he must be deluding himself. He was accepting of his medical colleagues and thought they genuinely believed that his observations could not be accurate. Unfortunately, seasoned researchers depending on government grants do not study adequate doses of vitamin C. This results in a massive accumulation of knowledge about little, which gives the impression that there is no more of real importance to be learned. This accumulation of minutia may hide the impressive effects of vitamin C that have been repeatedly reported and ignored.

levels and increased resistance to viral infection require the highest tolerable doses of vitamin C.

Dr. Cathcart gave vitamin C to bowel tolerance, which is the maximum
amount the body can take without causing diarrhea. Any person can
achieve this level for themselves. The bowel tolerance level is not a static
amount: *the sicker the patient, the more vitamin C their body needs and
will absorb.* As you return to health, you are not able to absorb as much,
and need to reduce the dose. The aim is to maintain an intake a little below
that which would cause loose bowels. It is a self-adjusting process.

Vitamin D

Vitamin D is called the "sunshine vitamin" because it can be made by the
skin in direct sunlight. In the body, vitamin D acts like a hormone and is
needed for bone health and immunity. Shortage of vitamin D is well
known to result in rickets, osteoporosis, and osteomalacia (bone thinning).
However, recent indications suggest deficiency of this nutrient is involved
in many additional conditions: high blood pressure,[43] cancer,[44] gum disease,[45] diabetes, atherosclerosis,[46] hip fracture in the elderly, and perhaps
dementia[47] are associated with shortage of vitamin D. Of particular interest is the effect on the immune system.

Ever wondered why people get colds and flu in winter rather than the
summer months? The body's levels of vitamin D are higher in the sunnier
months and decline in the winter. Similarly, multiple sclerosis occurs more
often in the more polar regions, rather than places near the equator. Vitamin D prevents bacterial and viral infections.[48] Claims for the benefits of
vitamin D supplementation are strong. An intake of several thousand IU
of vitamin D_3 a day will provide powerful immune support and may prevent a hospital-acquired infection. For full immune support, vitamin D_3
should be combined with high intakes of vitamin C.

Magnesium

The mineral magnesium is a catalyst for numerous biochemical reactions
in body cells. Along with calcium, magnesium is necessary for nerve function and muscular activity. Magnesium deficiency is common and can lead
to high blood pressure, heart disease, stroke, diabetes, and other chronic
conditions.[49] A long period of supplementation may be required to restore
healthy levels.[50] Try a twice daily dose of a chelated form, such as mag-

Preventing Bedsores

Bedsores are not an inevitable and necessary evil. Bedsores indicate poor nursing and hospital management. Sometimes called pressure ulcers, or decubitus ulcers, bedsores occur when the skin and underlying tissue are compressed for long periods. Other influences, such as shear force, friction, dampness, and temperature may contribute to forming or sustaining bedsores. Such sores are serious injuries: they extend from skin reddening, which does not fade when the pressure is relieved, to deep ulcers that can destroy muscle, tendon, or even bone. In severe bedsores, the bone may be visible. A typical bedsore can take many weeks to heal.[51] About half of all advanced bedsores heal within a year; however, treated conventionally, four out of ten bedsores never heal.

Bedsores are easily prevented by good nursing:

• Patients should turn or be turned every two hours

• Patients should be given heel pads to protect their feet

• Skin should be kept clean and dry

• Patients' skin should be examined regularly

• Daily patient skin care and massage should be routine

• Patients at risk may need pressure-reducing mattresses

One factor often overlooked in pressure sores is the role of nutrition. Bedsores do not just happen, they are allowed to happen. Inadequate hospital and nursing home food is a major culprit. Mild compression should not result in complete destruction of the tissues.

Bedsores might better be termed "scurvy sores" and, in centuries past, such ulcers often were. Scurvy, caused by shortage of vitamin C, results in bleeding gums and spontaneous pinpoint hemorrhaging. Small local areas of the skin and tissues are liable to spontaneous breakdown and bleeding. When it is short of vitamin C, the local tissue is unable to heal even the minor damage that normally occurs on a daily basis. Pressure and mechanical damage, from brushing the teeth or lying on a mattress, is enough to break blood vessels that are grossly weakened by a lack of vitamin C. The symptoms of acute scurvy include poor healing, weak capillaries, easy bruising, open wounds that suppurate (discharge pus), spontaneous bleeding, and internal hemorrhage, often from minor trauma. Descriptions of scurvy and of developing bedsores are remarkably similar.

Shortage of vitamin C has been considered a factor in the development and recovery from bedsores for many years.[52] Importantly, a person with bedsores may require several days of supplementation before their levels approach normal. In one study of patients with pressure sores, those treated with 500 mg of vitamin C a day recovered more quickly.[53] In the vitamin C group, the area of the sore reduced by 84 percent after one month; the control group had only half this recovery (42.7 percent reduction in area). More recent studies have confirmed the requirement for adequate vitamin C in association with supplemental arginine and zinc.[54]

Bedsores can be associated with severe inflammation and destruction of soft tissue and bone. Both share a number of symptoms, occur in malnourished patients, and are treatable with nutritional supplementation.[55] Vitamins C and B_3 (niacin) often work together, and this appears to be the case with bedsores. Pressure sores are a symptom of pellagra, a deficiency of niacin.[56] Back in 1946, it was reported that tropical ulcers were a symptom of vitamin B_3 deficiency, in American prisoners of war in the Philippines.[57] Niacin, the cure for pellagra, is also reported to help heal bedsores.[58]

Other nutrients will also be helpful. Zinc gluconate is readily available, cheap, and well-absorbed. A dose of 25 mg day of supplemental zinc is indicated. Vitamins A, B_1 (thiamine), B_2 (riboflavin), and E (natural mixed tocopherols or tocotrienols) are probably also helpful. Vitamin A and the B-vitamins can be found in any multivitamin preparation. The benefits to supplementing are improved healing, less discomfort, and reduced risk of infection and scarring. We should point out that Recommended Dietary Allowance (RDA) levels of nutrients, found in lower-quality supplements, are insufficient to prevent or help treat bedsores.[59]

Patients with bedsores and other chronic skin ulcers often have borderline malnutrition. Oral supplements will cover core nutrient requirements and their use in hospitalized elderly patients is justified.[60] Conservative treatment is preferred to surgery, and vitamin supplementation is about as conservative as it gets. Patients given optimal amounts of these nutrients will become more comfortable in days, although healing will take weeks.

> The amounts of vitamin C required to prevent bedsores and other disease are typically underestimated. Clinical claims for vitamin C relate to intakes above 10,000 mg a day, in divided doses. Once again, make sure you are taking dynamic flow doses of vitamin C, close to bowel tolerance level, which is just below the level that causes a laxative effect. An effective way to take vitamin C is to take the tablets several times a day, with each meal. Start with 500 mg with each meal (about every six hours) and increase the dose each day, until excessive wind or loose stools occur. The aim is to take just less than your maximum tolerated dose. Lower intakes are less likely to be effective.[61] The hospital and doctors may tell you it is unsafe. If so, make sure they provide a detailed explanation that is directly pertinent to your case. For example, it would be unwise to take high levels of vitamin C if a person had kidney disease or hemochromatosis (iron overload). However, in the absence of specific contraindications, there is little or no evidence that supplementing your diet is harmful.

nesium citrate. Read the label carefully to make sure you are getting about 200 mg of the element (magnesium) itself, not counting the accompanying molecule. The main side effect of overdose is loose stool. Avoid magnesium oxide supplements, which are particularly poorly absorbed.

WHEN YOU LEAVE THE HOSPITAL

Patients need to monitor their health and take precautions when they leave hospital after surgery.[62] The risk of a blood clot is increased seventy times in the six weeks after having surgery. For the twelve weeks following surgery, a person is at risk of developing deep vein thrombosis (DVT) or pulmonary embolism. These are potentially life-threatening problems of abnormal blood clotting. One in 140 middle-aged women will be readmitted with abnormal clotting within twelve weeks of surgery in hospital; these figures increase to one in forty-five after hip or knee replacement. Surgery for cancer is slightly safer in this respect, with one in eighty-five being readmitted. Surgery not requiring a hospital stay is safer still, with one in 815 suffering abnormal clots. Often, such readmissions will not be considered side effects of the original surgery.

After surgery, take action to prevent blood clots; remember to ask the doctor or nurse what precautionary measures you can take. Elastic stockings are available to help prevent DVT. Standing up, stretching and moving around will help. Ask what exercises are safe after your particular operation; if possible, take a short walk each day for the three months following the surgery.

There may be no clear symptoms with DVT. However, look out for:

• Discolored or visibly extended veins

• Pain, tenderness, or sudden swelling in one leg

• Skin that is unusually warm

Urgent assistance is needed if you have:

• Chest pain

• Shortness of breath

• Coughing blood

• Dizziness or fainting

• Disproportionate sweating

• Unusually rapid pulse

Patients can take nutrients that may help prevent such complications: as indicated previously, a gram (1,000 mg) or more of vitamin C three or four times a day, taken with fish oil, may help prevent DVT.

UNACCEPTABLE REASONS FOR STOPPING SUPPLEMENTATION

One of the most common issues with corporate medicine and particularly hospitals is their intolerance of vitamin supplementation. Sometimes, this prejudice can border on fanaticism. Here, we provide some specific advice for discussing supplementation as an example of using negotiation to get what you need.

• *"Vitamins will interfere with your tests."*—In response to the claim that vitamin supplementation can interfere with hospital tests, ask which tests are unreliable in this way. Do not expect a specific answer, however, as the data is unlikely to be available to the clinical staff making the claim. To answer this objection, ask for the phrase "takes supplements" to be added to any test paperwork. Remind them that everyone consumes vitamins in the diet as otherwise they would become sick. For any particular test, there will only be some supplements that are relevant. Ask which particular supplement will interfere with the test and why. Hospitals routinely have patients on several drugs at the same time without this interfering with their ability to perform and interpret diagnostic tests.

If there is a specific and essential test, or procedure, that requires suspension of a vitamin supplement, the particular vitamin can be stopped for a short period. The supplementation can be resumed immediately after the test is performed. Only a few supplements will need to be discontinued—those specifically known to interfere with the diagnostic test. Low-dose supplementation can continue, as vitamins and minerals are essential.

- *"Vitamins will be dangerous after surgery."*—There is a substantially increased need for vitamins and other nutrients during wound healing. For example, tissue repair requires synthesis of the structural protein collagen, for which vitamin C is needed. Some patients have been told that their blood-thinning medications, such as warfarin (Coumadin), are incompatible with vitamin supplements, especially vitamins K, C, and E. Vitamins C and E are essential to life. Vitamin C may lessen clotting time, and vitamin E may increase it, but it is not clear how a combination will influence the action of warfarin.

  The one vitamin supplement that is absolutely contraindicated with warfarin is vitamin K, as the drug specifically blocks its action. Warfarin is a vitamin K antagonist: blocking vitamin K produces its primary inhibition of blood clotting. The drug's action in blocking this vitamin also produces numerous side effects, including interactions with other drugs and dietary substances. Most people do not supplement with vitamin K and many multivitamins do not include this vitamin. Vitamin K is provided for the body by intestinal bacteria.

  The problems with warfarin are side effects of the drug, not nutrition. The use of this drug demands careful monitoring of blood clotting, typically at weekly to monthly intervals. The dose of the drug is adjusted to maintain a consistent clotting level. Use of supplements is entirely consistent with the use of warfarin, provided the drug is properly monitored and administered. We would not advise any dealings with a hospital that is unable to provide robust safe medication, monitoring, and control. Even warfarin can be combined with supplements.

• *"Vitamins are unnecessary on a normal diet."*—As indicated earlier, there is no evidence to support the oft-repeated statement that a normal diet provides all the nutrients necessary. This is an outdated idea from the early twentieth century, when it was thought that people only required micronutrients for good health. It is true that people get by living on burgers, chips, and other junk foods, but such a diet is unlikely to provide good health. The effects of a poor diet were graphically illustrated by Morgan Spurlock in his 2004 film *Super Size Me*. Most people in modern industrial societies have marginal nutritional deficiencies; for example, a large proportion of the population has low vitamin C and magnesium levels. It may be wise to ignore the statement that a normal diet provides all the nutrients necessary.

   The staff who claim that vitamin supplementation is unnecessary also carry some responsibility for the hospital food. Hospital food continues to deserve its almost pathogenic reputation.

If the Hospital Staff Remove Your Supplements

Hospital staff have *no* right to remove your vitamins or other supplements. They are your property. If they remove your supplements, demand they return them immediately. They have forced a negotiation.

Appeals to Authority

You are not a child and have the right to make decisions concerning your body. Accept nothing without an explanation that is satisfactory to you. If the nurse, doctor, aide, clerk, orderly, or anyone else makes a reference to authority, challenge the claim. It may be the hospital's rule, but who is the system intended to benefit? Ask for a supervisor. If the supervisor also claims that it is a rule, ask to see the hospital administrator. The rule should be backed up with a reason. Make it clear that they have a responsibility to you as a human being. If you are paying for your treatment, remind them. Remember, there are other hospitals and, unless your problem is acute, you can choose to leave.

SAFETY OF SUPPLEMENTS

Adverse drug side effects are a concern. Sick patients are often given multiple drugs and physicians end up treating the patient through a haze of side effects, and it is often impossible to tell what is the original disease or a side effect of an interacting drug. Still, doctors have an easier time than the patients.

While nutrition is accepted as a primary determinant of health, highlighting the potential dangers of supplements is routine in current medical papers reporting their benefits. This is ironic in an environment where adverse drug events are routinely accepted and an average hospital patient can expect to suffer at least one medication error per day. On the other hand, a review of poison control center reports reveals the amazing safety of vitamins.[63] The American Association of Poison Control Centers (AAPCC), which maintains the U.S. national toxicology database, indicates an extremely small number of deaths from vitamins in each given year. Keep in mind that these are national figures for an entire year.

ANNUAL DEATHS FROM VITAMINS			
YEAR	DEATHS	YEAR	DEATHS
2008	zero	1995	zero
2007	zero	1994	zero
2006	one	1993	one
2005	zero	1992	zero
2004	two	1991	two
2003	two	1990	one
2002	one	1989	zero
2001	zero	1988	zero
2000	zero	1987	one
1999	zero	1986	zero
1998	zero	1985	zero
1997	zero	1984	zero
1996	zero	1983	zero

This list includes the most recent data available at the time of writing.[64] The lack of deaths attributed to vitamins is not a result of selective coverage. AAPCC has noted that vitamins are among the sixteen most reported substances. Even including intentional and accidental misuse, the number of vitamin fatalities is strikingly low. In most years, the AAPCC reports that there was not one death due to vitamins. Plus, the causes of the reported deaths are typically not well determined and the risk may be an overestimate.

The safety of vitamin supplements is well established. The AAPCC data suggest an average risk of dying from vitamin supplementation in the U.S. to be less than one in 300 million a year; a person is at far greater risk of being struck by lightning. Despite this, a harmless niacin flush is often seen as sufficient justification to discontinue vitamin B_3 therapy for psychosis or cardiovascular disease. Some physicians declare that they simply do not "believe" in treating with vitamins but, unless one chooses to consult a shaman, such belief should have little to do with treatment.

Conclusion

Few people realize the danger that hospitals and medicine present to patients. Most people think of hospitals as high-technology cathedrals, where doctors save lives. In some cases, of course, hospitals are beneficial. Nevertheless, the horror story we have presented of medicine being a leading or even preeminent cause of death is not controversial. The hundreds of thousands of deaths that result from medical errors, mismanagement, or poor practice are recognized in the scientific press and apparently accepted by the wider public. Despite token attempts, there has been little effective action to prevent this slaughter.

Paying more for high-technology treatments may lead to greater harm. The Commonwealth Fund compared standards of health care in the United States with twelve other advanced countries: Australia, Canada, Denmark, England, France, Germany, Italy, The Netherlands, New Zealand, Norway, Sweden, and Switzerland.[1] The Netherlands, which topped the list, spent $3,837 per person a year on health care—less than half the spending by the bottom-placed U.S. ($7,290 per person a year). In the words of Karen Davis, president of the Commonwealth Fund, "As an American, it just bothers me that with all of our know-how, all of our wealth, that we are not assuring that people who need health care can get it."[2] Americans pay substantially more for a lower-quality, less-efficient medical system, which is unfair to patients. Until the philosophy, management, and control of medicine are updated, hospital patients need to reclaim responsibility for their own health.

Throughout much of their history, hospitals have been places that patients would have been well advised to avoid. Modern corporate medicine has an unprepossessing past. The scorned patent medicines of old

201

have fashioned modern pharmacy. Pharmaceutical companies and medical societies developed out of medieval guilds, designed to protect trade and professionals by creating monopolies. Nowadays, the main aim of drug companies is not to provide effective treatments but to maximize profits—indeed, this is a legal requirement for their company directors.

Descriptions of the terrible state of modern medicine are not new. In 1975, Ivan Illich explained how medical organizations were stealing our health for the benefit of corporations and professional physicians. Professions and organizations accumulate power, money, and influence primarily for their own benefit, not that of patients. Naturally, they try to acquire control and expand their importance. Their resulting monopolies have generated a licensed medical profession that excludes competing ideas and therapies. Such licensing is a relatively new phenomenon. However, do not be fooled into thinking the medical license exists to protect you from quacks; rather, it provides monopoly protection for the doctors. We see no evidence that the existence of medical licensing improves patient care. Despite all this regulation, many patients are still treated badly.

Doctors largely regulate themselves. They decide who is providing acceptable treatment and an implicit threat of deregistration for those who disagree or do not comply. The medical profession tends to avoid direct scientific comparison, but we would be surprised if nutritional and other "alternative" treatments did not provide superior results for the majority of patients. After this book's limited review of the catalog of medical failures, we hope the reader will be suspicious of the claims of conventional medicine and more open to the idea of improving health with alternatives. Nutritional medicine, in particular, claims to provide effective and safe treatments. Readers may take the opportunity to investigate for themselves.

The level of errors occurring in medicine would not be tolerated in other commercial fields. If a manufacturer produced an aircraft with even a small risk of falling out of the sky on each flight, people would simply refuse to use that plane. Similarly, a television manufacturer that did not provide a reliable, competitive product would rapidly lose market share. Corporate medicine fails its patients because it has legislated away the competition. The controls needed to reduce the risk of hospital death are simply not in place. The situation is so bad that the introduction of a straightforward checklist for surgery is seen as a major improvement. Hospitals and their staff are apparently so sure that they are helping people that they turn a blind eye to the contrary evidence.

The incidence of hospital infections is increasing and they are becoming untreatable by conventional medicine. In just a few decades, corporate medicine has destroyed the value of many antibiotics. To doctors who observed penicillin in the early days, it really was a miracle drug. Mismanagement and overuse means people now fear the resistant infections that are rampant in hospitals. Fortunately, for those with the time and inclination to investigate, high doses of vitamins C and D can provide a boost to host immunity, claimed to be at least the equivalent of the effects of early antibiotics. But do not expect to be offered such possibilities by corporate medicine—there is no money in it.

The loss of patients' rights is illustrated most sharply by the treatment of the mentally ill. Modern tranquilizing drugs are aptly named a "chemical cosh"—they interfere with and damp down the brain's function. With high doses, the patient can barely think or act at all, so it's no wonder they stop behaving and start talking strangely. Authorities have transferred psychiatric patients from locked wards and consigned many of them to a homeless life on the streets. There may be a better option for these people. Dr. Hoffer and others have described how high intakes of simple vitamins, such as niacin and vitamin C, might provide the basis for a successful treatment of schizophrenia. Corporate medicine offers long-term drug treatment, with chronic side effects and a life of dependency. By contrast, Dr. Hoffer reported a remarkably high rate of nutritional cure, which he defines as the patient returning to a useful and productive life.

Participative medicine is becoming the new paradigm: it is hoped that doctors will increasingly involve patients in decision making. However, current patients cannot expect medicine to reform itself in time for their next stay in the hospital. They can, however, take more control today. Doctors proposing a treatment should explain its potential benefits and risks fully. This book has explained briefly how the patient can view their interaction with health-care providers as a "game." Game theory suggests that a person should act to avoid the maximum risk. Strangely, if your health is in good condition, a health check-up may do more harm than good. For example, unless you have been at specific risk, a positive AIDS test may simply be misleading.

A rational person will value active good health, preventive medicine, and, particularly, supportive nutrition. If such a person needs treatment, they will treat it as a negotiation and make sure they are in charge. As the saying goes, everything is negotiable: you don't get what you deserve, you get what you negotiate!

Declaring a victory is an old ploy. Corporate medicine has claimed that, in the past, it provided benefits of extended life and freedom from disease. A closer examination of the data suggests that the eradication of the epidemic diseases of earlier centuries was mainly a result of improved sanitation and nutrition. The beneficial effects of medical interventions were secondary, if not irrelevant. Improved nutrition is usually given the credit for major increases in life expectancy and health. Likewise, poor nutrition is strongly implicated as a primary cause of the two predominant modern diseases of developed countries, cardiovascular disease and cancer. Indeed, the evidence suggests that our high levels of chronic disease, such as arthritis and late-onset diabetes, are also a result of chronic poor nutrition. This implies that earlier health improvements, attributed to improved nutrition, could continue into the future. Although corporate medicine considers this suggestion may be accurate, it campaigns vigorously against nutritional supplements.

Taking time to learn to get well and stay well is the most certain of investments. Sickness is expensive. Consider this: If you are pressed for time, but can spend some fraction of an hour each day improving your health, you will probably live longer. If you live longer, then you will have more time in the end. To keep control, we have to keep thinking, learning, and negotiating.

APPENDIX

Your Hospital Checklists

You want to leave the hospital on foot from the front door, not in a box by way of the basement. Take great care in choosing a hospital—your choice may save your life. In the United States, check out the Twelfth Annual HealthGrades Hospital Quality in America Study for the rating of your hospital.[1] The HealthGrades Study analyzed approximately 40 million Medicare discharges for quality as 1 star (poor), 3 stars (reasonable), and 5 stars (best). They compared twenty-seven procedures and diagnoses. In the three years from 2006 through 2008, they found a small improvement in mortality. Over seventeen procedures and diagnoses where death rates were studied, there was on average a 72 percent lower chance of dying in a highly rated hospital compared to a poor hospital. Compared with the average hospital, 5-star hospitals had less than half the risk of dying.

The report suggested that, from 2006 to 2008, 224,537 lives would be saved on Medicare if all hospitals had 5-star performance for the seventeen treatments. Over half of the preventable deaths were associated with four conditions: sepsis, pneumonia, heart failure, and respiratory failure. Remember that these statistics are people, with parents, wives, husbands, and children. Each of these deaths is a tragedy.

The results for complications were similar. While in the hospital for orthopedic procedures, there was an 80 percent lower chance of one or more complications if the hospital was 5-star rated hospital compared to a 1-star. The good hospitals were also much safer than the average ones. There was a 61 percent lower chance of one or more complications when in a 5-star rated hospital compared to the U.S. average. If all hospitals were working as well as a 5-star rated hospital, Medicare patients would have had 110,687 fewer orthopedic complications. Remember, a more expensive hospital is not necessarily safer. You need to select your hospital carefully.

Core Requirements for a Hospital

There are some core requirements for an institution attempting to heal the sick. The patient needs shelter, food, and respect. Unless these needs are met, there is little hope for effective treatment. However, patients may improve and get better in spite of the detrimental effects of the hospital.

The first requirement is to provide shelter. The failure of modern medicine in this respect is illustrated by the psychiatric patients begging on our streets. The patient needs shelter until well enough to carry on with his or her life outside the hospital.

The second requirement is for good nutritious food, and hospitals almost always fail on this. While it is generally accepted that much of modern disease is related to a poor diet, hospitals provide a terrible example in the food they typically serve. Do not expect the food you receive on a cardiology ward to adhere to the nutritional research on how to avoid a heart attack. Even when hospitals try to provide good nutrition, they are prevented by the current dietary paradigm. The majority of dietitians and nutritionists in hospitals are badly trained in vitamin therapy. As a rule, they promote vitamins and minerals only to the extent condoned by government standards such as the Recommended Dietary Allowance (RDA). Nutrition is perceived as part of preventive medicine and thus ignored by organizations dedicated to treatment. Some patients have their families bring them their meals, prepared at home from natural, fresh, whole foods—the classic grapes by the bedside. However, even an excellent diet does not provide sufficient nutrients to help heal serious illnesses. Supplements are essential.

The third factor is that patients need decency, respect, and optimism. Modern hospitals have much to learn from the Quaker model for mental hospitals.[2] The Quaker approach arose in the eighteenth century and the treatment included:

- Harmonious situation—building and surroundings that lift the spirit
- Nutrition—exceptional food standards
- Self-control—patients rewarded for controlling their behavior
- A return to socialization
- Useful work
- Staff as role models

The power of these simple requirements to aid recovery from psychiatric disorders is illustrated by the results claimed for schizophrenia by Dr. Hoffer and current medicine. Practitioners of orthomolecular and nutritional medicine necessarily provide good food and respect for the individual patient. The core element in Dr. Hoffer's treatment of schizophrenia was a very high intake of B vitamins, particularly niacin, and vitamin C. The reported recovery rates are shown in the table.

RECOVERY RATES FOR SCHIZOPHRENIA PATIENTS	
TREATMENT/ORGANIZATION	RECOVERY RATES
Mental hospital (1900 to 1950)	0 percent response
Modern psychiatry	Under 10 percent
Dr. Hoffer's orthomolecular treatment	75–90 percent

These figures are not directly challenged. When Dr. Hoffer reported them to colleagues, they suggested his excellent results were a result of his healing personality or self-delusion. Similarly, early critics of Dr. Hoffer's therapeutic clams never accused him of lying; instead, they provided alternative explanations, such as it was his amazing persona that was so beneficial. Dr. Hoffer was always the first to admit he really did have a marvelous personality, but he never considered it that powerful.

On one occasion, Dr. Hickey suggested a massive dose of niacin and vitamin C to a patient having an acute and severe psychotic episode. The young man was waiting for an appointment for mainstream psychiatric help. The results were immediate and dramatic: the young man recovered overnight and, within two days, had returned to normal. When he went for his appointment with the psychiatric services, he did not need medication or additional help. Dr. Hickey e-mailed Dr. Hoffer to tell him the news and received this tongue-in-cheek reply: "My critics never called me liar when I spoke about recoveries but they knew that it was due to my marvelous healing personality, as they also knew as a matter of fact that vitamins had absolutely nothing to do with schizophrenia. Now, we know that you too have that marvelous personality. Congratulations."

Here, we examine a number of factors you should look for in choosing a hospital and provide handy checklists to help your evaluation process.

BASIC CONSIDERATIONS

When choosing a hospital, there are a few basic considerations that may be helpful. Large hospitals and those connected to universities are more likely to have the equipment and expertise to cope in an emergency. However, take care with teaching hospitals—they are in need of material for research and training, and being a guinea pig is a risk you might want to avoid. Check that the hospital appears clean and well organized. Poor hospitals often have a bad reputation and this will be reflected in the opinion of former patients and perhaps local news reports. Do an Internet search on the hospital. Remember, you are far more likely to suffer complications or die in a poor hospital.

BASIC CONSIDERATIONS		
Is the hospital clean?	❏ Yes	❏ No
Are the corridors clear?	❏ Yes	❏ No
No bad smells?	❏ Yes	❏ No
Good staff/patient ratio?	❏ Yes	❏ No
Provides patient satisfaction forms?	❏ Yes	❏ No
Do care plan conferences include patients and relatives?	❏ Yes	❏ No
Friends and relatives provide positive reports?	❏ Yes	❏ No
Good reports in local press?	❏ Yes	❏ No
Are the nurses smiling?	❏ Yes	❏ No
Is it a large, well-provisioned hospital?	❏ Yes	❏ No
TOTAL SCORE:	_____ Yes	_____ No

An adequate hospital score is 8 of 10 or higher.

HOSPITAL WARDS/FLOORS

Checking hospital floors (wards) is straightforward. Look out for any breach of hygiene that will raise the risk of infection. The ward should be clean, welcoming, and well managed. Watch out for low numbers of nurses. In particular, make sure the hospital staff are focused on nutrition and have a positive attitude toward supplements. Ask about pressure sores—they should be rare or absent. Also, make sure that good food can be provided by relatives if the hospital food is poor. Arrange for a relative or friend to be with you throughout your stay.

HOSPITAL WARDS/FLOORS		
Are the rooms clean and tidy?	❏ Yes	❏ No
Nurses can monitor beds visually or are within calling distance?	❏ Yes	❏ No
The nurse/patient ratio is high?	❏ Yes	❏ No
Immediate response to calls for help and other requests?	❏ Yes	❏ No
Resuscitation and emergency equipment is immediately available?	❏ Yes	❏ No
Nurses are happy with staffing levels?	❏ Yes	❏ No
A patient will see a doctor each day?	❏ Yes	❏ No
Staff wash hands/change gloves between each patient?	❏ Yes	❏ No
A consulting physician controls all treatment?	❏ Yes	❏ No
Are cleaning staff visible and effective?	❏ Yes	❏ No
Staff report that there have been no recent issues with infection?	❏ Yes	❏ No
Nurses report normal supplies are at hand?	❏ Yes	❏ No
Food is excellent?	❏ Yes	❏ No
Nurses consider nutrition of primary importance?	❏ Yes	❏ No
Medical and nursing staff answer your questions politely and are helpful?	❏ Yes	❏ No
Are visitors welcome at any time?	❏ Yes	❏ No
TOTAL SCORE:	_____ Yes	_____ No

A score of 12 out of 16 is barely acceptable.

INFECTION CONTROL

One of the worst things about hospitals is that you can go into a hospital for surgery or another treatment and pick up an infection. As we have explained, this is more serious than it may sound. Hospital germs are often antibiotic-resistant "super-bugs."

INFECTION CONTROL		
Staff wash hands and change gloves between patients? Are you sure?	❏ Yes	❏ No
Are catheters cleaned regularly?	❏ Yes	❏ No
Ventilators are maintained regularly with the external airway changed each day?	❏ Yes	❏ No
Dressing changes are done with a sterile technique?	❏ Yes	❏ No
Waste needles, dressings, etc., are treated as biohazard waste?	❏ Yes	❏ No
Has the antibiotic been chosen as a result of a bacterial sensitivity test?	❏ Yes	❏ No
If the patient is in isolation, do the staff obey the same rules on masks, gowns, etc., as visitors?	❏ Yes	❏ No
TOTAL SCORE:	_____ Yes	_____ No

A score of 6 out of 7 is acceptable.

SAFE EMERGENCY ROOM?

In many cases, the choice of emergency department is moot. However, with minor injuries and conditions, it may be possible to have some flexibility over which emergency room (ER) you go to. Large hospitals have the imaging, intensive care, and other facilities necessary to properly support emergency medicine. Note that while an ER with a short waiting time is preferable, the imposition of target waiting times is a sign of poor management.

SAFE EMERGENCY ROOM?		
Is there a doctor for every ten patients?	❏ Yes	❏ No
Is there a nurse for every five patients?	❏ Yes	❏ No
Short waiting times?	❏ Yes	❏ No
Are security staff present?	❏ Yes	❏ No
Is the ER part of a large hospital?	❏ Yes	❏ No
TOTAL SCORE:	_____ Yes	_____ No

A score of 4 out of 5 is acceptable.

INTENSIVE CARE

Intensive is not necessarily beneficial. High-technology and "heroic" medicine is glamorous to the physician and makes exciting TV programs. Unless you have suffered major trauma, it is possible to have a long and full life without ever coming into contact with intensive medicine. As medicine becomes more intensive and invasive, it carries a correspondingly greater risk to the patient. All too often, patients need such intensive care because the hospital has made a life-threatening error. Try to stay with patients in intensive care, and check all their lines and procedures. The staff should be happy to explain what they are doing and why.

INTENSIVE CARE		
Is the patient monitored constantly?	❏ Yes	❏ No
There is a nurse for every three or fewer patients?	❏ Yes	❏ No
When you ask, you are told what each of the tubes and wires are for?	❏ Yes	❏ No
Where visible, the entry sites for intravenous (IV) drips are clean, not inflamed, swollen, reddened, or infected?	❏ Yes	❏ No
IV lines are dripping and have a drip chamber?	❏ Yes	❏ No
Blood from paid donors is not being used?	❏ Yes	❏ No
Are feeding tubes clean and the flow is acceptable?	❏ Yes	❏ No
The patient is not indicating problems with any tubes?	❏ Yes	❏ No
TOTAL SCORE:	_____ Yes	_____ No

A perfect score is necessary and is non-negotiable.

SURGERY

Elective or non-urgent surgery should be undertaken with clear knowledge of the risks and benefits. For example, is a straighter nose worth the financial cost and small risk of major loss of facial tissue through infection? Pre-surgery is one occasion where screening tests are appropriate. Before surgery, the patient should receive health checks, including blood cell counts and chemical analysis, clotting time, and an electrocardiogram (EKG). Try to ensure that there is someone in the recovery room at all times.

SURGERY		
Is the patient infection free?	❏ Yes	❏ No
Has the procedure been described in detail?	❏ Yes	❏ No
Have the possible complications been discussed?	❏ Yes	❏ No
Have the risks been identified and explained to you?	❏ Yes	❏ No
Will a suitably trained nurse be with you in the recovery room?	❏ Yes	❏ No
Does the operation have specific requirements for recovery?	❏ Yes	❏ No
High-dose vitamin C before and after the procedure?	❏ Yes	❏ No
TOTAL SCORE:	_____ Yes	_____ No

A score of 5 out of 7 is acceptable.

ANESTHESIA

A surgeon's mistake can cause you harm, disable you, or even kill you. However, it is even more critical to avoid an error by the anesthetist. One author suggests you ask the anesthetist to show his or her hand palm down and let you rest a sheet of paper on it.[3] He suggests you should request a different anesthetist if the hand is shaking.

ANESTHESIA		
Can you meet the anesthetist?	❏ Yes	❏ No
Is the anesthetist confident?	❏ Yes	❏ No
Does the anesthetist have at least five years of experience?	❏ Yes	❏ No
Does the anesthetist drink or smoke?	❏ Yes	❏ No
Will the anesthetist describe the process and the risks?	❏ Yes	❏ No
Does the anesthetist report a risk of death of at least one in 10,000?	❏ Yes	❏ No
Does the anesthetist give the impression that the procedure is routine?	❏ Yes	❏ No
TOTAL SCORE:	_____ Yes	_____ No

A score of 5 out of 7 is acceptable.

MOBILITY ISSUES

Patients with mobility issues have specific requirements. Falls in hospitals are a frequent cause of injury. Make sure everything needed is available and the patient does not need to leave the bed. Remember that following operations or other procedures, any patient can have mobility issues. Relatives of patients at risk who do not trust the hospital can help by visiting and monitoring the patient as much as possible.

MOBILITY ISSUES		
Is the patient unsteady on his or her feet?	❏ Yes	❏ No
Does the bed have side rails?	❏ Yes	❏ No
Is the nurse call switch within easy reach?	❏ Yes	❏ No
Are calls for assistance responded to immediately?	❏ Yes	❏ No
Do nurses make frequent patient checks both day and night?	❏ Yes	❏ No
Are water and other fluids within reach?	❏ Yes	❏ No
Are urinals and bedpans within reach?	❏ Yes	❏ No
Are patients told that assistance is available and they do not need to leave the bed?	❏ Yes	❏ No
Do the nurses appreciate the patient's risk?	❏ Yes	❏ No
If confusion is present, will the patient be monitored constantly day and night?	❏ Yes	❏ No
Is video surveillance in use?	❏ Yes	❏ No
TOTAL SCORE:	_____ Yes	_____ No

A score of 9 out of 11 is acceptable.

GIVING BIRTH

Hospitals are no safer than home births for normal deliveries, but they may be required if there are unusual health problems or risks. If having the baby at home, make sure you are prepared for a quick trip to the hospital in case of complications. Check the hospital's facilities and the route to be taken. Arrange for an ambulance to be available within five minutes to get the mother to hospital. The hospital should be large and well equipped to cover all eventualities.

The maternity unit needs to be secure. Hospitals make errors, such as operating on the wrong person or removing the wrong leg, so make sure you have the right baby! Check the nametag yourself and look for birthmarks as soon after birth as possible. Consider taking a footprint or handprint from the newborn or, better still, initial your baby's foot with an indelible marker. One of the authors (Andrew Saul) was almost switched in the hospital at his birth.

GIVING BIRTH		
Will fetal monitoring be employed and kept on throughout the birth?	❏ Yes	❏ No
Is a consulting obstetrician always available?	❏ Yes	❏ No
Does the hospital have full backup for emergencies, such as pediatric intensive care?	❏ Yes	❏ No
Is there a fully equipped crash cart nearby?	❏ Yes	❏ No
Is the unit secure?	❏ Yes	❏ No
How can the mother be sure the baby is not swapped accidentally?	❏ Yes	❏ No
Is the baby's heart rate between 100–160 beats per minute?	❏ Yes	❏ No
TOTAL SCORE:	_____ Yes	_____ No

A score of 5 out of 7 is adequate.

References

Introduction: Dangerous Places

1. Siegel-Itzkovich, J. "Doctors' Strike in Israel May Be Good for Health." *Br Med J* 320 (2000): 1561. Cunningham, S.A., K. Mitchell, K.M. Venkat Narayan, S. Yusu. "Doctors' Strikes and Mortality: A Review." *Social Sci Med* 67:11 (2008): 1784–1788.

2. Siegel-Itzkovich, J. "Doctors' Strike in Israel May Be Good for Health." *Br Med J* 320 (2000): 1561.

3. Steinherz, R. "Death Rates and the 1983 Doctors' Strike in Israel." *Lancet* 1:8368 (1984): 107.

4. Braly, J. "Doctor Strikes, Lowered Mortality—Happens Every Time." *BMJ Rapid Response* (March 5, 2000).

5. Laurance, J. "Health Check: During the Doctors' Strike in the 1970s, Death Rates Fell." *Independent Newspaper* (September 1, 2003).

6. Ostenson, R.M. "Striking Doctors Reduces Death Rates." *BMJ Rapid Response* (June 14, 2000).

7. Schimmel, E.M. "The Hazards of Hospitalization." *Qual Safe Health Care* 12 (2003): 58–63.

8. Steel, K., P.M. Gertman, C. Crescenzi, J. Anderson. "Iatrogenic Illness on a General Medical Service at a University Hospital." *N Engl J Med* 304 (1981): 638–642.

9. Gordon, R. *Great Medical Disasters*. London: Hutchinson, 1983.

10. Brit, R.R. "The Odds of Dying." Live Science. Livescience.com, (January 6, 2005).

11. Hayward, R.A., and T.P. Hofer. "Estimating Hospital Deaths Due to Medical Errors Preventability is in the Eye of the Reviewer." *JAMA* 286 (2001): 415–420.

12. McDonald, C.J., M. Weiner, S.L. Hui. "Deaths Due to Medical Errors are Exaggerated in Institute of Medicine Report." *JAMA* 284:1 (2000): 93–94.

13. Dubois, R.W., and R.H. Brook. "Preventable Deaths: Who, How Often, and Why?" *Ann Intern Med* 109 (1988): 582–589.

14. Kozak, L., and L. Lawrence. *National Hospital Discharge Survey: Annual Summary, 1997*. Hyattsville, MD: National Center for Health Statistics, 1999.

15. Andrews, L.B., C. Stocking, T. Krizek, et al. "An Alternative Strategy for Studying Adverse Events in Medical Care." *Lancet* 349 (1997): 309–313.

16. Null, G., C. Dean, M. Feldman, et al. "Death by Medicine." *Life Extension Magazine* (March 2004).

17. Wootton, D. *Bad Medicine: Doctors Doing Harm Since Hippocrates*. New York: Oxford University Press, 2007.

18. Gøtzsche, P.C., and O. Olsen. "Is Screening for Breast Cancer with Mammography Justifiable?" *Lancet* 355:9198 (2000):129–134.

19. List, S. "NHS is World's Biggest Employer after Indian Rail and Chinese Army." *Times Online* (March 20, 2004).

20. Ravnskov, U. *The Cholestrol Myths: Exposing the Fallacy That Saturated Fat and Cholesterol Cause Heart Disease*. Winona Lake, IN: New Trends Publishing, 2001.

21. Mendelsohn, R.S. *Confessions of a Medical Heretic*. New York: McGraw Hill, 1979.

22. Chan, P.S., H.M. Krumholz, G. Nichol, B.K. Nallamothu, and the American Heart Association National Registry of Cardiopulmonary Resuscitation Investigators. "Delayed Time to Defibrillation after In-Hospital Cardiac Arrest." *N Engl J Med* 358:1 (2008): 9–17.

23. Nordqvist, C. "Heart Attack in Casino Safer Than One in Hospital." *Medical News Today* (January 6, 2008).

24. Hippocrates. *Aphorisms*. Translated by Francis Adams. Massachusetts Institute of Technology, http://classics.mit.edu/Hippocrates/aphorisms.html. Accessed November 19, 2009.

25. Pear, R. "Study Finds Many Patients Dissatisfied with Hospitals." *The New York Times* (March 29, 2008).

26. Hickey, S., and A. Saul. *Vitamin C: The Real Story*. Laguna Beach, CA: Basic Health, 2008.

Chapter 1: How Did We Get Here?

1. Garrison, F.H. "The Evil Spoken of Physicians and the Answer Thereto." *Bull N Y Acad Med* 5:2 (1929): 145–156.

2. Strathern, P. *A Brief History of Medicine from Hippocrates to Gene Therapy*. London: Robinson, 2005.

3. Vadakan, M.D., and V. Vibul. "A Physician Looks at the Death of Washington." Early America Review, Archiving Early America. Earlyamerica.com. Accessed December 30, 2009.

4. Foucault, M. *The Birth of the Clinic: An Archaeology of Medical Perception*. New York: Vintage, 1994.

5. Wootton, D. *Bad Medicine: Doctors Doing Harm Since Hippocrates*. New York: Oxford University Press, 2007.

6. Nuland, S.B. *The Doctors' Plague: Germs, Childbed Fever, and the Strange Story of Ignác Semmelweis.* New York: W.W. Norton, 2004.

7. Kuhn, T. *The Structure of Scientific Revolutions.* Chicago: University of Chicago Press, 1996.

8. Sampson, W., and B.L. Beyerstein. "Traditional Medicine and Pseudoscience in China: A Report of the Second CSICOP Delegation (Part 2)." *Special Report* 20:5 (September/October 1996).

9. Chou, R., L.H. Huffman; American Pain Society; American College of Physicians. "Nonpharmacologic Therapies for Acute and Chronic Low Back Pain: A Review of the Evidence for an American Pain Society/American College of Physicians Clinical Practice Guideline." *Ann Intern Med* 147:7 (2007): 492–504.

10. Lee, A., Done M.L. "Stimulation of the Wrist Acupuncture Point P6 for Preventing Postoperative Nausea and Vomiting." *Cochrane Database Syst Rev* 3 (2004): CD003281.

11. Ezzo, J.M., M.A. Richardson, A. Vickers, et al. "Acupuncture-point Stimulation for Chemotherapy-induced Nausea or Vomiting." *Cochrane Database Syst Rev* 19:2 (2006): CD002285.

12. Melchart, D., K. Linde, P. Fischer, et al. "Acupuncture for Idiopathic Headache." *Cochrane Database Syst Rev* 1 (2001): CD001218.

13. Staud, R., and D.D. Price. "Mechanisms of Acupuncture Analgesia for Clinical and Experimental Pain." *Expert Rev Neurother* 6:5 (2006): 661–667.

14. Finger, S. *Origins of Neuroscience: A History of Explorations into Brain Function.* New York: Oxford University Press, 2001.

15. Saper, R.B., R.S. Phillips, A. Sehgal, et al. "Lead, Mercury, and Arsenic in U.S. and Indian-manufactured Ayurvedic Medicines Sold via the Internet." *JAMA* 300:8 (2008): 915–923.

16. Martena, M.J., J.C. Van Der Wielen, I.M. Rietjens, et al. "Monitoring of Mercury, Arsenic, and Lead in Traditional Asian Herbal Preparations on the Dutch Market and Estimation of Associated Risks." *Food Addit Contam Part A Chem Anal Control Expo Risk Assess* 27:2 (2010): 190–205.

17. Epstein, J., I.R. Sanderson, T.T. Macdonald. "Curcumin as a Therapeutic Agent: The Evidence from in Vitro, Animal and Human Studies." *Br J Nutr* 26 (2010): 1–13.

18. Moon, D.O., M.O. Kim, Y.H. Choi, et al. "Curcumin Attenuates Inflammatory Response in IL-1beta-induced Human Synovial Fibroblasts and Collagen-induced Arthritis in Mouse Model." *Int Immunopharmacol* 10:5 (2010): 605–610.

19. Harish, G., C. Venkateshappa, R.B. Mythri, et al. "Bioconjugates of Curcumin Display Improved Protection against Glutathione Depletion Mediated Oxidative Stress in a Dopaminergic Neuronal Cell Line: Implications for Parkinson's Disease." *Bioorg Med Chem* 18:7 (2010): 2631–2638.

20. Bar-Sela, G., R. Epelbaum, M. Schaffer. "Curcumin as an Anti-cancer Agent: Review of the Gap between Basic and Clinical Applications." *Curr Med Chem* 17:3 (2010): 190–197.

21. Angell, M. *The Truth About the Drug Companies*. New York: Random House, 2004.

22. Le Fanu, J. *The Rise and Fall of Modern Medicine*. Jackson, TN: Basic Books, 2002.

Chapter 2: Corporate Medicine and the Profit Motive

1. Angell, M. *The Truth About the Drug Companies*. New York: Random House, 2004.

2. Mendelsohn, R.S. *Confessions of a Medical Heretic*. New York: McGraw Hill, 1979.

3. Chapman-Smith, D. "Cost Effectiveness: The Manga Report." *The Chiropractic Report* (1993): 1–2.

4. Aetna Insurance Company. "The Managed Care Solution." Hartford, CT: Aetna Insurance, 1992, p. 2.

5. Epstein, S.R., and M. Prak. *Guilds: Innovation and the European Economy, 1400–1800*. Cambridge: Cambridge University Press, 2008.

6. Wiley, Harvey W. *The History of a Crime Against the Food Law*. Washington, DC: Harvey Wiley, 1929. Reprinted by the Lee Foundation for Nutritional Research, Milwaukee, WI, 1955.

7. U.S. Food and Drug Administration (FDA). *Defect Levels Handbook, The Food Defect Action Levels*. Bethesda, MD: U.S. Department of Health and Human Services, 2009.

8. Blaylock, R.L. *Excitotoxins: The Taste That Kills*. Sante Fe, NM: Health Press, 1996.

9. Angell, M. *The Truth About the Drug Companies*. New York: Random House, 2004. Kassirer, J.P. *On the Take: How Medicine's Complicity with Big Business Can Endanger Your Health*. New York: Oxford University Press, 2005.

10. Moynihan, R., and A. Cassels. *Selling Sickness: How the World's Biggest Pharmaceutical Companies are Turning Us All into Patients*. New York: Nation Books, 2006.

11. Picard, A. "Second Opinion: Tossing Out Leftover Drugs Costs Us in So Many Ways." *The Globe and Mail,* Toronto (March 23, 2006).

12. Comoretto, L., and S. Chiron. "Comparing Pharmaceutical and Pesticide Loads into a Small Mediterranean River." *Sci Total Environ* 349:1–3 (2005): 201–210.

13. Elliott, C. "The Drug Pushers." *The Atlantic* (April 2006): 82–93.

14. Leape, L.L., A.G. Lawthers, T.A. Brennan, W.G. Johnson. "Preventing Medical Injury." *QRB Qual Rev Bull* 19:5 (1993): 144–149. Brennan, T.A., L.L. Leape, N.M. Laird, et al. "Incidence of Adverse Events and Negligence in Hospitalized Patients. Results of the Harvard Medical Practice Study." *N Engl J Med* 324:6 (1991): 370–376.

15. Carvel, J. "Hundreds of Patients 'Died Unnecessarily' at Flagship Hospital." *The Guardian*. Guardian.co.uk (March 17, 2009).

16. Smith, R., and J. Bingham. "Failing Hospital: NHS Rating System Should Be Scrapped Says Inspection Chief." *Daily Telegraph,* telegraph.co.uk (November 27, 2009).

17. Silverman, W.A. "The Schizophrenic Career of a 'Monster Drug'." *Pediatrics* 110:2 Pt 1 (2002): 404–406.

18. Leape, L.L. "Institute of Medicine Medical Error Figures are Not Exaggerated." *JAMA* 284:1 (2000): 94–95.

19. Anderson, R.E., R.B. Hill, C.R. Key. "The Sensitivity and Specificity of Clinical Diagnostics During Five Decades: Toward an Understanding of Necessary Fallibility." *JAMA* 261 (1989): 1610–1617. Cameron, H.M., and E. McGoogan. "A Prospective Study of 1152 Hospital Autopsies, I: Inaccuracies in Death Certification." *J Pathol* 133 (1981): 273–283. Goldman, L., R. Sayson, S. Robbins, et al. "The Value of the Autopsy in Three Medical Eras." *N Engl J Med* 308 (1983): 1000–1005.

20. Prak, M.R., C. Lis, J. Lucassen (Editor), H. Soly. *Craft Guilds in the Early Modern Low Countries: Work, Power And Representation.* Farnham, England: Ashgate Publishing, 2006.

21. Illich, I. *Limits to Medicine: Medical Nemesis, the Expropriation of Health.* (Also known as *Medical Nemesis.*) London: Marion Boyars, 2000.

22. Ibid.

23. Ibid.

24. Appel, L.J., M.W. Brands, S.R. Daniels, et al.; American Heart Association. "Dietary Approaches to Prevent and Treat Hypertension: A Scientific Statement from the American Heart Association." *Hypertension* 47:2 (2006): 296–308.

25. Elliot, V.S. "Blood Pressure Readings Often Unreliable." American Medical Association, Amednews.com (June 11, 2007).

26. Jhalani, J., T. Goyal, L. Clemow, et al. "Anxiety and Outcome Expectations Predict the White-coat Effect." *Blood Press Monit* 10:6 (2005): 317–319.

27. Hickey, S., and H. Roberts. *Ascorbate: The Science of Vitamin C.* Morrisville, NC: Lulu Press, 2004.

28. Cochrane, A. *Effectiveness and Efficiency: Random Reflections on Health Services.* London: Nuffield Provincial Hospitals Trust, 1972.

29. Wootton, D. *Bad Medicine: Doctors Doing Harm Since Hippocrates.* New York: Oxford University Press, 2007.

30. McKeown, T. *The Modern Rise of Population.* New York: Academic Press, 1976.

31. Colgrove, J. "The McKeown Thesis: A Historical Controversy and Its Enduring Influence." *Am J Public Health* 92:5 (2002): 725–729.

32. Preston, S.H. "Population Studies of Mortality." *Population Stud* 50 (1996): 525–536.

33. Hollingsworth, T.H. (1964) "A Demographic Study of the British Ducal Families." *Population Stud* 18:Suppl (1964): 1–35. Wrigley, E.A., and R. Schofield. *The Population History of England 1541–1871: A Reconstruction.* Cambridge: Cambridge University Press, 1981.

34. Hodgart, R. (2009) "Schoolboy Wins Vitamin D Campaign." *Herald Scotland* (December 6, 2009).

35. Ward, J.W., and C. Warren. *Silent Victories: The History and Practice of Public Health in Twentieth-Century America.* New York: Oxford University Press, 2006.

36. Lieberman, T. "Do Doctors Always Tell the Truth? No, Reports the *Milwaukee Journal Sentinel.*" *Columbia Journal Rev* (November 13, 2009).

37. Miller, G.W. *King of Hearts: The True Story of the Maverick Who Pioneered Open Heart Surgery.* New York: Three Rivers Press, 2000.

38. Garrison, F.H. "The Evil Spoken of Physicians and the Answer Thereto." *Bull N Y Acad Med* 5:2 (1929): 145–156.

39. Burch, D. *Taking the Medicine.* London: Chatto & Windus, 2009.

Chapter 3: Poor Hospital Management

1. Lachmund, J. "Between Scrutiny and Treatment: Physical Diagnosis and the Restructuring of 19th Century Medical Practice." *Sociol Health Illness* 20:6 (2001): 779–801.

2. Southwick, A.F. "Hospital as an Institution—Expanding Responsibilities Change Its Relationship with the Staff Physician." 9 *Cal West L Rev* (1972–1973): 429.

3. Payne, W., and M. Pflanz. "One in Five HIV Infections Caused by Medical Staff: One in Five HIV Sufferers in Africa was Infected by Medical Staff Using Dirty Needles and Clinical Equipment, New Research has Found." *London Telegraph,* telegraph.co .uk (November 30, 2009).

4. Reid, S., and A.A. Van Niekerk. "Injection Risks and HIV Transmission in the Republic of South Africa." *Int J Sex Transmit Dis AIDS* 20 (2009): 816–819.

5. Reid, S. "Non-vertical HIV Transmission to Children in Sub-Saharan Africa." *Int J Sex Transmit Dis AIDS* 20 (2009): 820–827.

6. Hunsmann, M. "Political Determinants of Variable Aetiology Resonance: Explaining the African AIDS Epidemics." *Int J Sex Transmit Dis AIDS* 20 (2009): 834–838.

7. Gisselquist, D. "Double Standards in Research Ethics, Health-care Safety, and Scientific Rigour Allowed Africa's HIV/AIDS Epidemic Disasters." *Int J Sex Transmit Dis AIDS* 20 (2009): 839–845.

8. Vincent, J.L., J. Rello, J. Marshall, et al. "International Study of the Prevalence and Outcomes of Infection in Intensive Care Units." *JAMA* 302:21 (2009): 2323–2329.

9. Ibid.

10. Cooper, H., G. Findlay, A.P.L. Goodwin, et al. *Caring to the End? A Review of the Care of Patients Who Died in Hospital within Four Days of Admission.* London: National Confidential Enquiry into Patient Outcome and Death, 2009.

11. Ibid.

12. Devlin, K. "Poor Care 'Could Be Killing Patients'." *London Telegraph,* telegraph .co.uk (November 22, 2009).

13. World Health Organization (WHO). "Definition of Palliative Care." WHO, who.int/cancer/palliative/definition/en/; accessed November 22, 2009.

14. Hill, A. "NHS 'is Lacking Humanity', says Catholic Leader." *The Observer* (February 14, 2010).

15. Schneider, J.A. "Qualified Privilege for Peer Review: Physician, Reveal Thyself." 17 *Pac L J* (1985–1986): 499.

16. Appel, J.M. "Must My Doctor Tell My Partner? Rethinking Confidentiality in the HIV Era." *Med Health R I* 89:6 (2006): 223–224.

17. Von Kanel, R.L. "Confidentiality—An Analysis of the Issue." *Plast Surg Nurs* 17:3 (1997): 146–147; 154–155.

18. Erlen, J.A. "The Inadvertent Breach of Confidentiality." *Orthop Nurs* 17:2 (1998): 47–50. Erlen, JA. "How Confidential is Confidential?" *Orthop Nurs* 27:6 (2008): 357–360.

19. Gladwell, M. *Outliers: The Story of Success.* New York: Penguin, 2009.

20. Gunderman, R., and M. Cohen. "Why Planes Crash: Lessons for Radiology." *J Am Coll Radiol* 6:7 (2009): 518–520.

21. Merritt, A. "Replicating Hofstede: A Study of Pilots in Eighteen Countries." In: Jensen, R.S. (ed.). *Proceedings of the Ninth International Symposium on Aviation Psychology.* Columbus, OH: Ohio State University, 1998, 667–672.

22. Merritt, A.C. "Culture in the Cockpit: Do Hofstede's Dimensions Replicate?" *J Cross-Cultural Psych* 31:3 (2000): 283–301. Merritt, A., and R.L. Helmreich. "Human Factors on the Flight Deck: The Influence of National Culture." *J Cross-Cultural Psych* 27:1 (1996): 5–24.

23. Goss, M.E.W. "Influence and Authority Among Physicians in an Outpatient Clinic." *Am Sociol Rev* 26:1 (1961): 39–50.

24. Chase, S.K. "The Social Context of Critical Care Clinical Judgment." *Heart Lung* 24:2 (1995): 154–162.

25. Album, D., and S. Westin. "Do Diseases have a Prestige Hierarchy? A Survey Among Physicians and Medical Students." *Soc Sci Med* 66:1 (2008): 182–188.

26. Lerner, B.H. "In a Hospital Hierarchy, Speaking Up is Hard To Do." *The New York Times* (April 17, 2007).

27. Schmid Mast, M. "Dominance and Gender in the Physician–Patient Interaction." *J Men's Health Gender* 1:4 (2004): 354–358.

28. Milgram, S. *Obedience to Authority: An Experimental View.* New York: Harper Collins, 1974.

29. Hofling, C.K., E. Brotzman, S. Dalrymple, et al. "An Experimental Study in Nurse–Physician Relationships." *J Nerv Mental Dis* 143:2 (1966): 171–180.

30. U.S. Food and Drug Administration (FDA). "Computed Tomography (CT)." U.S. Food and Drug Administration, fda.gov. accessed February 15, 2010.

31. MacLean, C.D. "Principles of Cancer Screening." *Med Clin North Am* 80:1 (1996): 1–14.

32. Greenemeier, L. "Hospital Error Leads to CT Scan Radiation Overdoses in 206 Patients." *Sci Am Health Med* (October 13, 2009).

33. U.S. Food and Drug Administration (FDA). "Safety Investigation of CT Brain Perfusion Scans, Initial Notification." Issued: October 8, 2009.

34. Ballantyne, C. "Can a Simple Checklist Prevent Surgical Errors?" *Sci Am Health Med* (January 14, 2009).

35. Harmon, K. "Deaths from Avoidable Medical Error More than Double in Past Decade, Investigation Shows." *Sci Am Health Med* (August 10, 2009).

36. Anonymous. "Boeing 747-400, by the Numbers." Boeing, Inc., boeing.com. Accessed November 27, 2009.

37. Deming, W.E. *Out of the Crisis,* 2nd ed. Cambridge, MA: MIT Press, 2000.

38. Sack, K. "Doctors Say 'I'm Sorry' Before 'See You in Court'." *The New York Times* (May 18, 2008).

39. Asthana, A. (2005) "Try Saying Sorry, NHS Doctors Told." *The Observer* (September 18, 2005).

40. Taxis, K., and N. Barber. "Ethnographic Study of Incidence and Severity of Intravenous Drug Errors." *Br Med J* 326 (2003): 684–687.

41. Breyfogle, F.W. *Business Deployment, Vol. II: A Leaders' Guide for Going Beyond Lean Six Sigma and the Balanced Scorecard: 2 (Integrated Enterprise Excellence).* Austin, TX: Bridgeway Books, 2008.

Chapter 4: A Look at Hospital-Acquired Infections

1. Weinstein, R.A. "Nosocomial Infection Update. Special Issue." *Emerg Infect Dis* 4:3 (1998).

2. Null, G., and M. Feldman. *Death by Medicine.* Edinburg, VA: Praktikos Books, 2010.

3. Maxwell-Lyte, H.C. *The Register of Thomas Bekynton, Bishop of Bath and Wells 1443-1465, Vol. 49.* Somerset, UK: Somerset Record Society, 1934.

4. Carlin, M. "Medieval English Hospitals." In Granshaw, L., and R. Porter (eds.). *The Hospital in History.* London: Routledge, 1989. Noskin, G.A., and L.R. Peterson. (2001) "Engineering Infection Control through Facility Design." *Emerg Infect Dis* 7:2 (March-April 2001): 354–357.

5. Hoyt, E.P. *The Improper Bostonian: Dr. Oliver Wendell Holmes.* New York: Morrow, 1979.

6. Chesney, A.M. *The Johns Hopkins Hospital and the Johns Hopkins University School of Medicine.* Baltimore: Johns Hopkins Press, 1943.

7. Bacon, A.S. "Efficient Hospitals." *JAMA* 74 (1920): 123–126.

8. American Institute of Architects. *Guidelines for Design and Construction of Hospital and Health Care Facilities, 1996–97.* Washington, DC: American Institute of Architects Press, 1996.

9. Doebbeling, B.N., M.A. Ishak, B.H. Wade, et al. "Nosocomial Legionella micdadei Pneumonia: 10 Years Experience and a Case-control Study." *J Hosp Infect* 13:3 (1989): 289–298.

10. Jasmer, R.M., P. Nahid, P.C. Hopewell. "Clinical Practice. Latent Tuberculosis Infection." *N Engl J Med* 347:23 (2002): 1860–1866.

11. Dolin, P.J., M.C. Raviglione, A. Kochi. "Global Tuberculosis Incidence and Mortality During 1990–2000." *Bull WHO* 72:2 (1994): 213–220.

12. Chan, T.Y.K. "Vitamin D Deficiency and Susceptibility to Tuberculosis." *Calcif Tiss Int* 66:6 (2000): 476–478. Also: Chocano-Bedoya, P., and A.G. Ronnenberg. "Vitamin D and Tuberculosis." *Nutr Rev* 67:5 (May 2009): 289–293. Martineau, A.R., R.J. Wilkinson, K.A.Wilkinson, et al. "A Single Dose of Vitamin D Enhances Immunity to Mycobacteria." *Am J Respir Crit Care Med* 176:2 (July 2007): 208–213.

13. Rotter, M.L. "150 Years of Hand Disinfection—Semmelweis' Heritage." *Hygiene Med* 22 (1997): 332–339.

14. Gould, D. "Hand-washing: Can Ward-based Learning Improve Infection Control?" *Nurs Times* 92:24 (1996): 42–43.

15. Pritchard, V., and C. Hathaway. "Patient Handwashing Practice." *Nurs Times* 84:36 (1988): 68–72.

16. Bartzokas, C.A., E.E. Williams, P.D. Slade. "A Psychological Approach to Hospital-acquired Infections." In *Studies in Health and Human Sciences*. London: Edward Mellen, 1995.

17. Tibballs, J. "Teaching Hospital Medical Staff to Handwash." *Med J Aust* 164:7 (1996): 395–398.

18. Handwashing Liaison Group. "Hand Washing, A Modest Measure with Big Effects." (Editorial.) *Br Med J* 318 (1999): 686–686.

19. Weeks, W. "Why I Don't Wash My Hands Between Each Patient Contact." *Br Med J* 319 (1999): 518.

20. Kesavan, S. "Handwashing Facilities are Inadequate." *Br Med J* 319 (1999): 518.

21. Heenan, A. "Hand Washing Practices." *Nurs Times* 88 (1992): 69–70.

22. MacDermott, R. "Dermatitis Associated with Frequent Hand Washing Should Have Been Mentioned." *Br Med J* 319 (1999): 518.

23. Marinella, M.A., C. Pierson, C. Chenoweth. "The Stethoscope. A Potential Source of Nosocomial Infection?" *Arch Intern Med* 157 (1997): 786–790.

24. Wong, D., K. Nye, P. Hollis. "Microbial Flora on Doctors' White Coats." *Br Med J* 303 (1991): 1602–1604.

25. Kesavan, S., S. Barodawala, G.P. Mulley. "Now Wash Your Hands? A Survey of Hospital Handwashing Facilities." *J Hosp Infect* 40 (1998): 291–293.

26. Perry, J., G. Parker, J. Jagger. "EPINet Report: 2007 Percutaneous Injury Rates." Charlottesville, VA: International Healthcare Worker Safety Center, August 2009.

27. Delamothe, T. "Everything You Know is Wrong." *Br Med J* 337 (2008): a3027.

28. Rosenberg, C. "Florence Nightingale. Reputation and Power, by Smith F.B., Review by Charles Rosenberg." *Med Hist* 27:1 (1983): 93.

29. Williams, K. "Reappraising Florence Nightingale." *Br Med J* 337 (2008): a2889.

30. Gordon, R. *Great Medical Disasters.* London: Scutari, Hutchinson, 1983.

31. Nightingale, F. *Notes on Hospitals.* London: John W. Parker & Son, 1859.

32. Smith, F.B. *Florence Nightingale: Reputation and Power.* London: Croom Helm, 1982.

33. Attewell, A. "Florence Nightingale 1820–1910." *Prospects Qtr Rev Compar Educ* 18:1 (1998): 153–166.

34. Nightingale, F. *Notes on Nursing: What It Is, And What It Is Not.* New York: D. Appleton, 1898.

35. Halliday, S. "Death and Miasma in Victorian London: An Obstinate Belief." *Br Med J* 323 (2001): 1469–1471.

36. Neuhauser, D. "Heroes and Martyrs of Quality and Safety: Florence Nightingale Gets No Respect: As a Statistician That Is." *Qual Safe Health Care* 12 (2003): 317.

37. Pain, S. "Histories: The 'Male' Military Surgeon Who Wasn't." *New Sci* (March 6, 2008).

38. Kubba, A.K. "The Life, Work and Gender of Dr. James Barry, MD (1795–1865)." *Proc R Coll Physicians Edinb* 31 (2001): 352–356.

39. Neuhauser, D. "Heroes and Martyrs of Quality and Safety: Florence Nightingale Gets No Respect: As a Statistician That Is." *Qual Safe Health Care* 12 (2003): 317.

40. McCabe, P. "Naturopathy, Nightingale, and Nature Cure: A Convergence of Interests." *Complement Ther Nurs Midwifery* 6:1 (2000): 4–8.

41. Seacole, M. *Wonderful Adventures of Mrs. Seacole in Many Lands.* London: James Blackwood, 1857.

42. Morozumi, S. "Isolation, Purification, and Antibiotic Activity of o-Methoxycin-namaldehyde from Cinnamon." *Appl Environ Microbiol* 36:4 (1978): 577–583. Kalemba, D., and A. Kunicka. "Antibacterial and Antifungal Properties of Essential Oils." *Curr Med Chem* 10:10 (2003): 813–829. Shan, B., Y.Z. Cai, J.D. Brooks, H. Corke. "Antibacterial Properties and Major Bioactive Components of Cinnamon Stick (*Cinnamomum burmannii*): Activity Against Foodborne Pathogenic Bacteria." *J Agric Food Chem* 55:14 (2007): 5484–5490.

43. Rutala, W.A., E.B.S. Katz, R.J. Sherertz, F.A. Sarubbi Jr. "Environmental Study of a Methicillin-resistant *Staphylococcus aureus* Epidemic in a Burn Unit." *J Clin Microbiol* 18 (1983): 683–688.

44. Livornese, L.L., S. Dias, C. Samel, et al. "Hospital-acquired Infection with Vancomycin-resistant *Enterococcus faecium* Transmitted by Electronic Thermometers." *Ann Intern Med* 117:2 (1992): 112–116.

45. Kaatz, G.W., S.D. Gitlin, D.R. Schaberg, et al. "Acquisition of *Clostridium difficile* from the Hospital Environment." *Am J Epidemiol* 127:6 (1988): 1289–1294.

46. U.S. Centers for Disease Control and Prevention (CDC). "Antibiotic/Antimicrobial Resistance." CDC, http://www.cdc.gov/drugresistance/, 2008. U.S. Centers for Disease Control and Prevention (CDC). "Get Smart: Know When Antibiotics Work." CDC, http://www.cdc.gov/GetSmart/antibiotic-use/fast-facts.html.

47. Arias, C.A., and B.E. Murray. "Antibiotic-Resistant Bugs in the 21st Century—A Clinical Super-Challenge." *N Engl J Med* 360:5 (2009): 439–443.

48. Null, G., C. Dean, M. Feldman, D. Rasio. "Death by Medicine." *J Orthomolecular Med* 20:1 (2005): 21–34.

49. Egger, W.A. "Antibiotic Resistance: Unnatural Selection in the Office and on the Farm." *Wisconsin Med J* 101:5 (2002): 12–13.

50. Shehab, N., P.R. Patel, A. Srinivasan, D.S. Budnitz. "Emergency Department Visits for Antibiotic-associated Adverse Events." *Clin Infect Dis* 47:6 (2008): 735–743.

51. Ibid.

52. Arrigo, G., and A. D'Angelo. "Achromycin and Anaphylactic Shock." *Riv Patol Clin* 14 (1959): 719–722. Harvey, H.P., and H.J. Solomon. "Acute Anaphylactic Shock Due to Para-aminosalicylic Acid." *Am Rev Tubercul* 77:3 (1958): 492–495. Lythcott, G.I. "Anaphylaxis to Viomycin." *Am Rev Tubercul* 75:1 (1959): 135–138. Farber, J.E., J. Ross, G. Stephens. "Antibiotic Anaphylaxis." *Calif Med* 81:1 (1954): 9–11. Farber, J.E., and J. Ross. "Antibiotic Anaphylaxis; A Note on the Treatment and Prevention of Severe Reactions to Penicillin, Streptomycin and Dihydrostreptomycin." *Med Times* 80:1 (1952): 28–30. Patterson, D.B. "Anaphylactic Shock from Chloromycetin." *Northwest Med* 49:5 (1950): 352–353.

53. Cathcart, R.F. "Vitamin C, Titration to Bowel Tolerance, Anascorbemia, and Acute Induced Scurvy." *Med Hypotheses* 7 (1981): 1359–1376.

54. Saul, A.W. "The Pioneering Work of William J. McCormick, M.D." *J Orthomolecular Med* 18:2 (2003): 93–96. Klenner, F.R. "The Use of Vitamin C as an Antibiotic." *J Appl Nutr* 6 (1953): 274–278.

55. McCormick, W.J. "Ascorbic Acid as a Chemotherapeutic Agent." *Arch Pediatrics NY* 69:4 (1952): 151–155.

56. Ayliffe, G.A.J., B.J. Collins, E.J.L. Lowbury, et al. "Ward Floors and Other Surfaces as Reservoirs of Hospital Infection." *J Hygeine* 65 (1967): 515–536.

Chapter 5: Psychiatry and the Limits of Modern Medicine

1. Conolly, J. *An Inquiry Concerning the Indications of Insanity, with Suggestions for the Better Protection and Care of the Insane 1794–1866*. London: Taylor, 1830.

2. Rosenhan, D.L. "On Being Sane in Insane Places." *Science* 179:70 (1973): 250–258.

3. Spitzer, R.L. "More on Pseudoscience in Science and the Case for Psychiatric Diagnosis." *Arch Gen Psychiatry* 33:4 (1976): 459–470.

4. Slater, L. *Opening Skinner's Box: Great Psychological Experiments of the Twentieth Century*. New York: W.W. Norton, 2005.

5. Hoffer, A. *Healing Children's Attention and Behavior Disorders*. Toronto, ON, Canada: CCNM Press, 2005.

6. Adams, J. (1977) "Orthomolecular Psychiatry." *Cosmopolitan* (June 1997).

7. Milgram, S. "Behavioral Study of Obedience." *J Abnorm Soc Psych* 67 (1963): 371–378.

8. Tierney, J. "Diet and Fat: A Severe Case of Mistaken Consensus." *The New York Times* (October 9, 2007).

9. Asch, S.E. "Opinions and Social Pressure." *Sci Am* 193 (1955): 31–35.

10. Safire, W. "The Way We Live Now: Groupthink." *The New York Times* (August 8, 2004).

11. Alexander, S.P. "Unusual Fracture of the Pelvis Due to ECT." *Psychiatric Qtr* 28:1 (1954): 613–615.

12. Parsons, W.B., Jr. *Cholesterol Control Without Diet: The Niacin Solution.* Scottsdale, AZ: Lilac Press, 2003.

13. Stevens, L. "Psychiatric Drugs: Cure or Quackery?" whale.to/a/stevens1.html. Accessed December 23, 2009.

14. Madsen, A.L., N. Keiding, A. Karle, et al. "Neuroleptics in Progressive Structural Brain Abnormalities in Psychiatric Illness." *Lancet* 352 (1998): 784–785.

15. Strathern, P. *A Brief History of Medicine.* London: Robinson, 2005.

16. Lieberman, J.A., T.S. Stroup, J.P. McEvoy, et al. "Effectiveness of Antipsychotic Drugs in Patients with Chronic Schizophrenia." *N Engl J Med* 353 (2005): 1209–1223.

17. Triggle, N. "Dementia 'Chemical Cosh' Warning." BBC News (November 12, 2009).

18. Boseley, S. "Care Homes Forcing Elderly to Have Feeding Tubes Fitted." *The Guardian* (January 6, 2010).

19. Carey, B. "Revisiting Schizophrenia: Are Drugs Always Needed?" *The New York Times* (March 21, 2006).

20. Leighton, R., R.P. Feynman, E. Hutchings. *Surely You're Joking, Mr. Feynman!: Adventures of a Curious Character.* New York: Vintage, 1992.

21. Aldhous, P. "Psychiatry's Civil War." *New Sci* (December 11, 2009).

22. Frances, A. "A Warning Sign on the Road to DSM-V: Beware of Its Unintended Consequences." *Psychiatric Times* (June 26, 2009).

23. Frances, A. "DSM 5 Goes Too Far in Creating New Mental Disorders: Holding the Line between Normality and Mental Disorder." *Psychology Today* (March 10, 2010).

24. Conolly, J. *An Inquiry Concerning the Indications of Insanity, with Suggestions for the Better Protection and Care of the Insane 1794–1866.* London: Taylor, 1830.

25. Hoffer, A., H. Kelm, H. Osmond. *The Hoffer-Osmond Diagnostic Test.* Huntington, NY: R.E. Krieger, 1975. The HOD Test Kit is available (in English only) from Behavior Science Press, Institute for Social and Educational Research, 3710 Resource Drive, Tuscaloosa AL 35401-7059.

26. Ward, P.E., J. Sutherland, E.M. Glen, A.I. Glen. "Niacin Skin Flush in Schizophrenia: A Preliminary Report." *Schizophr Res* 29:3 (1998): 269–274.

27. Bosveld-van Haandel, L., R. Knegtering, H. Kluiter, R. van den Bosch. "Niacin Skin Flushing in Schizophrenic and Depressed Patients and Healthy Controls." *J Psychiatry Res* 143:2–3 (2006): 303–306.

28. Liu, C.M., S.S. Chang, S.C. Liao, et al. "Absent Response to Niacin Skin Patch is Specific to Schizophrenia and Independent of Smoking." *Psychiatry Res* 152:2–3 (2007): 181–187. Chang, S.S., C.M. Liu, S.H. Lin, et al. "Impaired Flush Response to Niacin Skin Patch Among Schizophrenia Patients and Their Nonpsychotic Relatives: The Effect of Genetic Loading." *Schizophr Bull* 35:1 (2009): 213–221.

29. Hoffer, A. "Chronic Schizophrenic Patients Treated Ten Years or More." *J Orthomolecular Med* 9 (1994): 7–37.

30. Williams, S.R. *Nutrition and Diet Therapy,* 6th edition. New York: Times Mirror/Mosby, 1989.

31. Hoffer, A., H. Kelm, H. Osmond. *The Hoffer-Osmond Diagnostic Test.* Huntington, NY: R.E. Krieger, 1975. The HOD Test Kit is available (in English only) from Behavior Science Press, Institute for Social and Educational Research, 3710 Resource Drive, Tuscaloosa AL 35401-7059.

32. Hoffer A., Saul A.W. *Orthomolecular Medicine for Everyone: Megavitamin Therapeutics for Families and Physicians.* Laguna Beach, CA: Basic Health Publications, 2008.

Chapter 6: The Hospital Game

1. Haug, M.R. "A Re-examination of the Hypothesis of Physician Deprofessionalization." *Milbank Q* 66:Suppl 2 (1988): 48–56.

2. Brett, J.M. *Negotiating Globally: How to Negotiate Deals, Resolve Disputes, and Make Decisions Across Cultural Boundaries.* San Francisco: Jossey-Bass, 2007.

3. von Neumann, J., O. Morgenstern, with A. Rubinstein, H.W. Kuhn. *Theory of Games and Economic Behavior.* Princeton, NJ: Princeton University Press, 2007.

4. Atkinson, R. "NHS Power Games." [Letters.] *The Daily Mail* (May 7, 2009).

5. Leape, L.L. "Unnecessary Surgery." *Annu Rev Public Health* 13 (1992): 363–383.

6. Kelman, C.W., M.A. Kortt, N.G. Becker, et al. "Deep Vein Thrombosis and Air Travel: Record Linkage Study." *Br Med J* 327 (2003): 1072.

7. Heit, J.A., M.D. Silverstein, D.N. Mohr, et al. "Risk Factors for Deep Vein Thrombosis and Pulmonary Embolism: A Population-based Case-control Study." *Arch Intern Med* 160:6 (2000): 809–815.

8. Lifeblood. "About Thrombosis." Thrombosis_charity.org. Accessed May 12, 2009.

9. McManus, A. "Preventing a Blood Clot When in Hospital." Lifeblood, The Thrombosis Charity Report, October 2007.

10. All-Party Parliamentary Thrombosis Group. "Thrombosis: Awareness, Assessment, Management and Prevention, Second Annual Audit of Acute NHS Hospital Trusts." London: United Kingdom government report, November 2008.

11. Walton, M. *The Trouble with Medicine: Preserving the Trust Between Patients and Doctors.* St. Leonards, NSW, Australia: Allen & Unwin, 1998.

12. Starr, P. *The Social Transformation of American Medicine: The Rise of a Sovereign Profession and the Making of a Vast Industry.* New York: Basic Books, 1984.

13. Pellegrino, E.D., and D.C. Thomasma. *The Virtues in Medical Practice.* New York: Oxford University Press, 1994.

14. BBC News. "Hospital Phobia Woman Ordered to Have Surgery." BBC, bbc.co.uk (May 27, 2010). Accessed May 28, 2010.

15. Martin, D. "Judge Forces Patient with Hospital Phobia to Have Lifesaving Cancer Surgery." Mail Online, *The Daily Mail,* dailymail.co.uk (May 27, 2010). Accessed May 28, 2010.

16. Beckford, M., S. Adams, L. Roberts. (2010) "Woman with Hospital Phobia Must Be Forcibly Treated for Cancer, Judge Rules." *The Daily Telegraph,* telegraph.co.uk (May 26, 2010). Accessed May 30, 2010.

17. Aschner, M., and J.L. Aschner. "Mercury Neurotoxicity: Mechanisms of Blood–Brain Barrier Transport." *Neurosci Biobehav Rev* 14:2 (1990): 169–176.

18. Newman, M.F., J.L. Kirchner, B. Phillips-Bute, et al.; Neurological Outcome Research Group and the Cardiothoracic Anesthesiology Research Endeavors Investigators. "Longitudinal Assessment of Neurocognitive Function after Coronary-artery Bypass Surgery." *N Engl J Med* 344:6 (2001): 395–402.

19. Fogoros, R.N. "Pump Head—Cognitive Impairment after Bypass Surgery." About.com Guide, November 28, 2003. Accessed February 6, 2010. Fogoros, R.N. (2004–2009) "Pump Head—Not a Problem After All? New Study Casts Doubt on Seriousness of Post-CABG Dementia." About.com Guide. Accessed February 6, 2010.

20. Samuels, M.A. "Can Cognition Survive Heart Surgery?" *Circulation* 113:24 (2006): 2784–2786.

21. Miller, A.B., and J. Linseisen. "Achievements and Future of Nutritional Cancer Epidemiology." *Int J Cancer* 126:7 (2010): 1531–1537.

22. George, D.R., A.D. Dangour, L. Smith, et al. "The Role of Nutrients in the Prevention and Treatment of Alzheimer's Disease: Methodology for a Systematic Review." *Eur J Neurol* 16:Suppl 1 (2009): 8–11.

23. Pollan, S.M., and M. Levine. *The Total Negotiator.* New York: Avon Books, 1994.

24. Shell, G.R. *Bargaining for Advantage: Negotiation Strategies for Reasonable People.* New York: Penguin, 2006.

25. Fisher, R., B.M. Patton, W.L. Ury. *Getting to Yes: Negotiating Agreement Without Giving In.* Boston: Houghton Mifflin, 1992.

26. Tang, H., and J.H.K. Ng. "Googling for a Diagnosis—Use of Google as a Diagnostic Aid: Internet Based Study." *Br Med J* 333 (2006): 1143–1145.

27. Freund, J.C. *Smart Negotiating: How to Make Good Deals in the Real World.* New York: Simon & Schuster, 1993.

28. PDR Staff. *Physicians' Desk Reference 2008,* Hospital/Library Version, 62nd ed. Oradell, NJ: Medical Economics, 2007.

29. Martin, J. *British National Formulary,* 55th ed. London: Pharmaceutical Press, 2007.

Chapter 7: Take Charge of Your Health Care

1. Mongerson, P. "A Patient's Perspective of Medical Informatics." *J Am Med Inform Assoc* 2 (1995): 79–84.

2. Blendon, R.J., C.M. DesRoches, M. Brodie, et al. "Views of Practicing Physicians and the Public on Medical Errors." *N Engl J Med* 347 (2002): 1933–1940.

3. YouGov Survey of Medical Misdiagnosis, 2005. Isabel Healthcare-Clinical Decision Support System. Reported by Berner, E.S., and M.L. Graber. "Overconfidence as a Cause of Diagnostic Error in Medicine." *Am J Med* 121:5 Suppl (2008): S2–S23.

4. Berner, E.S., and M.L. Graber. "Overconfidence as a Cause of Diagnostic Error in Medicine. *Am J Med* 121:5 Suppl (2008): S2–S23.

5. Fitzgerald, R. "Error in Radiology." *Clin Radiol* 56 (2001): 938–946.

6. Kronz, J.D., W.H. Westra, J.I. Epstein. "Mandatory Second Opinion Surgical Pathology at a Large Referral Hospital." *Cancer* 86:11 (1999): 2426–2435.

7. Kripalani, S., M.V. Williams, K. Rask. "Reducing Errors in the Interpretation of Plain Radiographs and Computed Tomography Scans." In: Shojania, K.G., et al. *Making Health Care Safer: A Critical Analysis of Patient Safety Practices.* Rockville, MD: Agency for Healthcare Research and Quality, 2001. Available online at: http://archive.ahrq.gov/clinic/tp/ptsaftp.htm#Report.

8. Gigerenzer, G. *Calculated Risks: How to Know When Numbers Deceive You.* New York: Simon & Schuster, 2003.

9. Gigerenzer, G., and P.M. Todd; ABC Research Group. *Simple Heuristics That Make Us Smart.* New York: Oxford University Press, 2000.

10. Neale, G., M. Woloshynowych, C. Vincent. "Exploring the Causes of Adverse Events in NHS Hospital Practice." *J R Soc Med* 94 (2001): 322–330.

11. Williams, R. *Biochemical Individuality.* New York: McGraw-Hill, 1998.

12. Chellis, M., J. Olson, J. Augustine, G. Hamilton. "Evaluation of Missed Diagnoses for Patients Admitted from the Emergency Department." *Acad Emerg Med* 8 (2001): 125–130.

13. O'Connor, P.M., K.E. Dowey, P.M. Bell, et al. "Unnecessary Delays in Accident and Emergency Departments: Do Medical and Surgical Senior House Officers Need to Vet Admissions?" *Accid Emerg Med* 12:4 (1995): 251–254.

14. Berner, E.S., and M.L. Graber. "Overconfidence as a Cause of Diagnostic Error in Medicine. *Am J Med* 121:5 Suppl (2008): S2–S23.

15. Gould, S. J. "The Median isn't the Message." *Discover* (June 6, 1985): 40–42.

16. Sutherland, S. *Irrationality.* London: Pinter & Martin, 2007.

17. Hickey, S., and H. Roberts. *Cancer: Nutrition and Survival.* Morrisville, NC: Lulu Press, 2007.

18. Chapman, J.A., N.A. Miller, H.L. Lickley, et al. "Ductal Carcinoma in Situ of the Breast (DCIS) with Heterogeneity of Nuclear Grade: Prognostic Effects of Quantitative Nuclear Assessment." *BMC Cancer* 7 (2007): 174.

19. Eddy, D. "Probabilistic Reasoning in Clinical Medicine: Problems and Opportunities. In: Kahneman, D., P. Slovic, A. Tversky. *Judgment Under Uncertainty: Heuristics and Biases.* Cambridge, England: Cambridge University Press, 1982.

20. Sutherland, S. *Irrationality.* London: Pinter & Martin, 2007.

21. Wooton, D. *Bad Medicine: Doctors Doing Harm Since Hippocrates.* New York: Oxford University Press, 2006.

22. Gigerenzer, G. *Calculated Risks: How to Know When Numbers Deceive You.* New York: Simon & Schuster, 2003.

23. Brennan, T.A., A. Gawande, E. Thomas, D. Studdert. "Accidental Deaths, Saved Lives, and Improved Quality." *N Engl J Med* 353:13 (2005): 1405–1409.

24. McCannon, C.J., M.W. Schall, D.R. Calkins, A.G. Nazem. "Saving 100,000 Lives in U.S. Hospitals." *Br Med J* 332 (2006): 1328–1330.

25. Berwick, D.M., D.R. Calkins, J. McCannon, A.D. Hackbarth. "The 100,000 Lives Campaign, Setting a Goal and a Deadline for Improving Health Care Quality." *JAMA* 295 (2006): 324–327. Hackbarth, A.D., C.J. McCannon, D.M. Berwick. "Interpreting the 'Lives Saved' Result of IHI's 100,000 Lives Campaign." *Jt Comm Benchmark* 8:5 (2006): 1–11.

26. Tanne, J.H. "U.S. Campaign to Save 100,000 Lives Exceeds Its Target." *Br Med J* 332:7556 (2006): 1468.

27. Trossman, S. "Campaign Meets and Exceeds Goal of Saving 100,000 Lives." *Am Nurse* 38:4 (2006): 1–10.

28. Sandrick, K. "Quality Exponential: The Journey from 100,000 to 5 Million Lives." *Trustee* 60:10 (2007): 14–16.

29. McCannon, C.J., A.D. Hackbarth, F.A. Griffin. "Miles to Go: An Introduction to the 5 Million Lives Campaign." *Jt Comm J Qual Patient Safety* 33:8 (2007): 477–484.

30. Wachter, R.M., and P.J. Pronovost. "The 100,000 Lives Campaign: A Scientific and Policy Review." *Jt Comm J Qual Patient Safety* 32:11 (2006): 621–627.

31. Ross, T.K. "A Second Look at 100,000 Lives Campaign." *Qual Manag Health Care* 18:2 (2009): 120–125.

32. World Health Organization (WHO). "Global Tuberculosis Control, WHO Report 2009." WHO, http://www.who.int/tb/publications/global_report/2009/en/index.html, 2009.

33. Kumar, V., A.K. Abbas, N. Fausto, R.M. Robbins. *Basic Pathology,* 8th ed. Philadelphia: Elsevier, 2007.

34. Cannell, J.J., R. Vieth, J.C. Umhau, et al. "Epidemic Influenza and Vitamin D." *Epidemiol Infect* 134:6 (2006): 1129–1140.

35. Wilkins, L., and C.P. Richter. "A Great Craving for Salt by a Child with Corticoadrenal Insufficiency." *JAMA* 114 (1940): 866–868.

36. Weir, J.S. "Chemical Properties and Occurrence on Kalahari Sand of Salt Licks Created by Elephants." *J Zool* 158:3 (1969): 293–310.

37. Newton, P., and N. Wolfe. "Can Animals Teach Us Medicine?" *Br Med J* 305:6868 (1992): 1517–1518.

38. Serpell, J. *The Domestic Dog: Its Evolution, Behaviour and Interactions with People.* Cambridge, England: Cambridge University Press, 1995.

39. Kirk, C.A., J. Debraekeleer, P.J. Armstrong. "Normal Cats." In: *Small Animal Clinical Nutrition,* 4th ed. Topeka, KS: Mark Morris Institute, 2000.

40. Phillips-Conroy, J.E. "Baboons, Diet and Disease: Food Selection and Schistosomiasis." In: Taub, D.M., and F.A. King (eds.). *Current Perspective in Primate Social Dynamics.* New York: Van Nostrand Reinhold, 1986.

41. Newton, P., and T. Nishida. "Possible Buccal Administration of Herbal Drugs by Wild Chimpanzees (*Pan troglodytes*)." *Animal Behav* 139 (1990): 799–800.

42. Walker, M. "Wild Orangutans Treat Pain with Natural Anti-inflammatory." *New Sci* 28 (July 2008).

43. Morrogh-Bernard, H.C. "Fur-Rubbing as a Form of Self-Medication in *Pongo pygmaeus.*" *Int J Primatol* 29:4 (2008): 1059–1064.

44. Eysenbach, G. "Medicine 2.0: Social Networking, Collaboration, Participation, Apomediation, and Openness." *J Med Internet Res* 10:3 (2008): e22.

45. Giustini, D. "How Web 2.0 is Changing Medicine." *Br Med J* 333 (2006): 1283–1284.

46. Crespo, R. "Virtual Community Health Promotion." *Prev Chronic Dis* 4:3 (2007): A75.

47. Tang, H., and J.H. Ng. "Googling for a Diagnosis—Use of Google as a Diagnostic Aid: Internet Based Study." *Br Med J* 333:7579 (2006): 1143–1145.

48. Surowieki, J. *The Wisdom of Crowds.* New York: Anchor, 2005.

49. Murray, E., B. Lo, L. Pollack, et al. "The Impact of Health Information on the Internet on Health Care and the Physician–Patient Relationship: National U.S. Survey Among 1050 U.S. Physicians." *J Med Internet Res* 5:3 (2003): e17.

50. Anonymous. "Health 2.0: Technology and Society: Is the Outbreak of Cancer Videos, Bulimia Blogs and Other Forms of 'User Generated' Medical Information a Healthy Trend?" *The Economist* (September 6, 2007): 73–74

51. Ojalvo, H.E. "Online Advice: Good Medicine or Cyber-quackery?" American College of Physicians, acponline.org/journals/news/dec96/cybrquak.htm. Accessed December 28, 2009.

52. Sutherland, S. *Irrationality.* London: Pinter & Martin, 2007.

53. Wald, N.J., and M.R. Law. "A Strategy to Reduce Cardiovascular Disease by More than 80 Percent." *Br Med J* 326:7404 (2003): 1419.

54. Dickinson, A., N. Boyon, A. Shao. (2009) "Physicians and Nurses Use and Recommend Dietary Supplements: Report of a Survey." *Nutr J* 8 (2009): 29–36.

Chapter 8: The Power of Nutrition

1. Brennan, C. "Vitamin Supplements: Good or Bad?" NetDoctor.com. http://www.net-doctor.co.uk/menshealth/feature/vitamins.htm.

2. Taylor, A.J., T.C. Villines, E.J. Stanek, et al. "Extended-Release Niacin or Ezetimibe and Carotid Intima-Media Thickness." *N Engl J Med* 361:22 (2009): 2113–2122.

3. Peck, P. "Zetia Fails to Show Benefit Over Niacin for Heart Patients. Cheap Vitamin B Beats Pricier Cholesterol Drug in Clearing Arteries." *MedPage Today,* ABC News, Orlando, FL, November 16, 2009.

4. British Medical Association, Royal Pharmaceutical Society of Great Britain. *British National Formulary,* 58. London: Pharmaceutical Press, 2009.

5. Bjelakovic, G., D. Nikolova, R.G. Simonetti, C. Gluud. "Antioxidant Supplements for Prevention of Gastrointestinal Cancers: A Systematic Review and Meta-analysis." *Lancet* 364 (2004): 1219–1227.

6. Roberts, L.J., J.A. Oates, M.F. Linton, et al. "The Relationship between Dose of Vitamin E and Suppression of Oxidative Stress in Humans." *Free Radic Biol Med* 43:10 (2007): 1388–1393.

7. The Alpha-Tocopherol, Beta Carotene Cancer Prevention Study Group. "The Effect of Vitamin E and Beta Carotene on the Incidence of Lung Cancer and Other Cancers in Male Smokers." *N Engl J Med* 330:15 (1994): 1029–1035. Omenn, G.S., G. Goodman, M. Thornquist, et al. "The Beta-carotene and Retinol Efficacy Trial (CARET) for Chemoprevention of Lung Cancer in High Risk Populations: Smokers and Asbestos-exposed Workers." *Cancer Res* 54:7 Suppl (1994): 2038s–2043s.

8. Lee, I.M., N.R. Cook, J.E. Manson. "Beta-carotene Supplementation and Incidence of Cancer and Cardiovascular Disease: Women's Health Study." *J Natl Cancer Inst* 91 (1999): 2102–2106. Hennekens, C.H., J.E. Buring, J.E. Manson, et al. "Lack of Effect of Long-term Supplementation with Beta Carotene on the Incidence of Malignant Neoplasms and Cardiovascular Disease." *N Engl J Med* 334 (1996): 1145–1149.

9. Ioannidis, J.P.A. "Why Most Published Research Findings are False." *PLoS Med* 2:8 (2005): e124.

10. Bjelke, E. "Dietary Vitamin A and Human Lung Cancer." *Int J Cancer* 15:4 (1975): 561–565.

11. Michael, P. "Possible Cancer Cure Found in Blushwood Shrub." *Courier Mail* (February 4, 2010), CourierMail.com.au, accessed February 12, 2010.

12. Ecobiotics. "First Cancer Drug from the Australian Rainforest to Enter Human Clinical Trials." As seen on "A Current Affair," Press release, October 22, 2009.

13. Hickey, S., and H. Roberts. *Cancer: Nutrition and Survival.* Morrisville, NC: Lulu Press, 2005.

14. Goldstein, A. "Child Hunger an Increasingly Complex Problem." *Washington Post* (December 12, 2009).

15. Wilson, D. "Poor Children Likelier to Get Antipsychotics." *The New York Times* (December 11, 2009). Crystal, S., M. Olfson, C. Huang, et al. "Broadened Use of Atyp-

ical Antipsychotics: Safety, Effectiveness, and Policy Challenges." *Health Affairs* 28:5 (2009): w770–w781.

16. Wachs, T.D. "Models Linking Nutritional Deficiencies to Maternal and Child Mental Health." *Am J Clin Nutr* 89:3 (2009): 935S–939S.

17. Ames, B.N. "DNA Damage from Micronutrient Deficiencies is Likely To Be a Major Cause of Cancer." *Mutat Res* 475:1–2 (2001): 7–20.

18. Marinacci, B. (ed.). *Linus Pauling in His Own Words: Selections from His Writings, Speeches, and Interviews.* New York: Simon and Shuster, 1995

19. Stone, I. *The Healing Factor: Vitamin C Against Disease.* New York: Grosset and Dunlap, 1972. The text of this book is posted online at: http://vitamincfoundation .org/stone.

20. Ridker, P.M., E. Danielson, F.A.H. Fonseca, et al., for the JUPITER Study Group. "Rosuvastatin to Prevent Vascular Events in Men and Women with Elevated C-Reactive Protein." *N Engl J Med* 359:21 (2008): 2195–2207.

21. Smith, R. "Millions Could Cut Heart Attack Risk by Taking Statins, Study Finds." *London Telegraph,* telegraph.co.uk (November 10, 2008).

22. Hope, J. "The New Statin Drug that Cuts the Risk of Heart Attacks and Strokes for Everyone." *Daily Mail* (November 11, 2008).

23. Devaraj, S., R. Tang, B. Adams-Huet, et al. "Effect of High-dose Alpha-tocopherol Supplementation on Biomarkers of Oxidative Stress and Inflammation and Carotid Atherosclerosis in Patients with Coronary Artery Disease." *Am J Clin Nutr* 86:5 (2007): 1392–1398.

24. Block, G., C.D. Jensen, T.B. Dalvi, et al. "Vitamin C Treatment Reduces Elevated C-reactive Protein." *Free Radic Biol Med* 46 (2009): 70–77. Sardi, B. "The Headline You Should Be Reading: Statin Drugs Don't Save Lives and May Increase Your Risk for Diabetes." *Knowledge of Health Report* (November 11, 2008).

25. Law, M., and A.R. Rudnicka. "Statin Safety: A Systematic Review." *Am J Cardiol* 97:8 Suppl 1 (2006): S52–S60.

26. Ridker, P.M.; JUPITER Study Group. "Rosuvastatin in the Primary Prevention of Cardiovascular Disease among Patients with Low Levels of Low-density Lipoprotein Cholesterol and Elevated High-sensitivity C-reactive Protein: Rationale and Design of the JUPITER Trial." *Circulation* 108:19 (2003): 2292–2297.

27. Ford, E.S., S. Liu, D.M. Mannino, et al. "C-reactive Protein Concentration and Concentrations of Blood Vitamins, Carotenoids, and Selenium among United States Adults." *Eur J Clin Nutr* 57 (2003): 1157–1163.

28. Root, M.M., J. Hu, L.S. Stephenson, et al. "Determinants of Plasma Retinol Concentrations of Middle-aged Women in Rural China." *Nutrition* 15 (1999): 101–107.

29. Boosalis, M.G., D.A. Snowdon, C.L. Tully, M.D. Gross. "Acute Phase Response and Plasma Carotenoid Concentrations in Older Women: Findings from the Nun Study." *Nutrition* 12 (1996): 475–478.

30. Friso, S., P.F. Jacques, P.W. Wilson, et al. "Low Circulating Vitamin B(6) is Asso-

ciated with Elevation of the Inflammation Marker C-reactive Protein Independently of Plasma Homocysteine Levels." *Circulation* 103:23 (2001): 2788–2791. Devaraja, S., and I. Jialal. "Alpha Tocopherol Supplementation Decreases Serum C-reactive Protein and Monocyte Interleukin-6 Levels in Normal Volunteers and Type 2 Diabetic Patients." *Free Radical Biol Med* 29:8 (2000): 790–792. Upritchard, J.E., W.H. Sutherland, J.I. Mann. "Effect of Supplementation with Tomato Juice, Vitamin E, and Vitamin C on LDL Oxidation and Products of Inflammatory Activity in Type 2 Diabetes." *Diabetes Care* 23 (2000): 733–738.

31. Ioannidis, J.P.A. "Why Most Published Research Findings are False." *PLoS Med* 2:8 (2005): e124.

32. Chandra, R.K. "Nutrition and Immunity: Basic Considerations, Part 1." *Contemp Nutr* 11:11 (1986): 1–2.

33. Patterson, B.H., G. Block, W.F. Rosenberger, et al. "Fruit and Vegetables in the American Diet: Data from the NHANES II Survey." *Am J Public Health* 80 (1990): 1443–1449.

34. Alexander, M., H. Newmark, R.G. Miller. "Oral Beta-carotene Can Increase the Number of OKT4+ Cells in Human Blood." *Immunol Lett* 9:4 (1985): 221–224.

35. Cohen, B.E., G. Gill, P.R. Cullen, P. Morris. "Reversal of Postoperative Immunosuppression in Man by Vitamin A." *J Surg Gynecol Obstet* 149:5 (1979): 658–662.

36. Hickey, S., and H. Roberts. *Ascorbate: The Science of Vitamin C.* Morrisville, NC: Lulu Press, 2004.

37. Williams, S. *Nutrition and Diet Therapy,* 7th ed. Philadelphia: Mosby, 1989.

38. Werbach, M.R. *Nutritional Influences on Illness.* New Canaan, CT: Keats Publishing, 1988.

39. Klenner, F.R. "Virus Pneumonia and its Treatment with Vitamin C." *S Med Surg* (February 1948): 36–46.

40. Pauling, L. *How to Live Longer and Feel Better.* New York: W.H. Freeman, 1986.

41. Cathcart, R.F. "Vitamin C in the Treatment of Acquired Immune Deficiency Syndrome." *Med Hypotheses* 14 (1984): 423–433.

42. Brighthope, I., and P. Fitzgerald. *The AIDS Fighters.* New Canaan, CT: Keats Publishing, 1988.

43. Pilz, S., A. Tomaschitz, E. Ritz, T.R. Pieber. "Vitamin D Status and Arterial Hypertension: A Systematic Review." *Nat Rev Cardiol* 6:10 (2009): 621–630.

44. Pilz, S., A. Tomaschitz, B. Obermayer-Pietsch, et al. "Epidemiology of Vitamin D Insufficiency and Cancer Mortality." *Anticancer Res* 29:9 (2009): 3699–3704.

45. Amano, Y., K. Komiyama, M. Makishima. "Vitamin D and Periodontal Disease." *J Oral Sci* 51:1 (2009): 11–20 .

46. Melamed, M.L., P. Muntner, E.D. Michos, et al. "Serum 25-Hydroxyvitamin D Levels and the Prevalence of Peripheral Arterial Disease: Results from NHANES 2001 to 2004." *Arterioscler Thromb Vasc Biol* 28:6 (2008): 1179–1185.

47. Grant, W.B. "Does Vitamin D Reduce the Risk of Dementia?" *J Alzheimers Dis* 17:1 (2009): 151–159. Llewellyn, D.J., K.M. Langa, I.A. Lang. "Serum 25-Hydroxyvitamin D Concentration and Cognitive Impairment." *J Geriatr Psychiatry Neurol* 22:3 (2009): 188–195.

48. Adams, J.S., P.T. Liu, R. Chun, et al. "Vitamin D in Defense of the Human Immune Response." *Ann N Y Acad Sci* 1117 (2007): 94–105.

49. Seeling, M., and A. Rosanoff. *Magnesium Factor.* New York: Avery Publishing, 2003.

50. Dean, C. *The Magnesium Miracle.* New York: Ballantine Books, 2006.

51. Thomas, D.R., M.R. Diebold, L.M. Eggemeyer. "A Controlled, Randomized, Comparative Study of a Radiant Heat Bandage on the Healing of Stage 3–4 Pressure Ulcers: A Pilot Study." *J Am Med Dir Assoc* 6:1 (2005): 46–49.

52. [No Authors Listed.] "Ascorbic Acid and Pressure Sores." *Br Med J* 2:5762 (1971): 604–605.

53. Taylor, T.V., S. Rimmer, B. Day, et al. "Ascorbic Acid Supplementation in the Treatment of Pressure-sores." *Lancet* 2:7880 (1974): 544–546.

54. Desneves, K.J., B.E. Todorovic, A. Cassar, T.C. Crowe. "Treatment with Supplementary Arginine, Vitamin C and Zinc in Patients with Pressure Ulcers: A Randomised Controlled Trial." *Clin Nutr* 24:6 (2005): 979–987. Frías Soriano, L., M.A. Lage Vázquez, C.P. Maristany, et al. "The Effectiveness of Oral Nutritional Supplementation in the Healing of Pressure Ulcers." *J Wound Care* 13:8 (2004): 319–322.

55. Buchanan, J.A.G., M. Cedro, A. Mirdin, et al. "Necrotizing Stomatitis in the Developed World." *Clin Exp Dermatol* 31:3 (2006): 372–374.

56. Roberts, S.R. *Pellagra: History, Distribution, Diagnosis, Prognosis, Treatment, Etiology.* St. Louis: Mosby, 1912. Cumbee, L. "The Nursing Care of Pellagra." *Am J Nurs* 31:3 (1931): 272–274.

57. Lewis, C.F., and M.M. Musselman. "Observations on Pellagra in American Prisoners of War in the Philippines." *J Nutr* (July 1946): 549–558.

58. Gernand, K. "Therapy of Ulcus Cruris and Decubitus." *Dtsch Gesundheitspolit* 6:48 (1951): 1388–1389.

59. Selvaag, E., T. Bøhmer, K. Benkestock. "Reduced Serum Concentrations of Riboflavin and Ascorbic Acid, and Blood Thiamine Pyrophosphate and Pyridoxal-5-phosphate in Geriatric Patients with and without Pressure Sores." *J Nutr Health Aging* 6:1 (2006): 75–77. Powers, J.S., J. Zimmer, K. Meurer, et al. "Direct Assay of Vitamins B_1, B_2, and B_6 in Hospitalized Patients: Relationship to Level of Intake." *J Parenter Enteral Nutr* 17:4 (1993): 315–316.

60. Raffoul, W., M.S. Far, M.C. Cayeux, M.M. Berger. "Nutritional Status and Food Intake in Nine Patients with Chronic Low-limb Ulcers and Pressure Ulcers: Importance of Oral Supplements." *Nutrition* 22:1 (2006): 82–88.

61. ter Riet, G., A. Kessels, P. Knipschild. "Randomized Clinical Trial of Ascorbic Acid in the Treatment of Pressure Ulcers." *J Clin Epidemiol* 48:12 (1995): 1453–1460.

62. Sweetland, S., J. Green, B. Liu, et al. "Duration and Magnitude of the Postoperative Risk of Venous Thromboembolism in Middle Aged Women: Prospective Cohort Study." *Br Med J* 339 (2009): b4583.

63. American Association of Poison Control Centers (AAPCC). Annual Reports of the American Association of Poison Control Centers' National Poisoning and Exposure Database (formerly known as the Toxic Exposure Surveillance System). Washington, DC: AAPCC, 1983–2009.

64. Bronstein, A.C., D.A. Spyker, L.R. Cantilena Jr., et al. "Annual Report of the American Association of Poison Control Centers' National Poison Data System (NPDS), 26th Annual Report." *Clin Toxicol* 47 (2008): 911–1084.

Conclusion

1. Squires, D.; the Commonwealth Fund, and Others. International Profiles of Health Care Systems: Australia, Canada, Denmark, England, France, Germany, Italy, The Netherlands, New Zealand, Norway, Sweden, Switzerland, and the United States. New York: The Commonwealth Fund, June 23, 2010.

2. Fox, M. "U.S. Scores Dead Last Again in Healthcare Study." Reuters News Service, Washington, D.C., June 23, 2010.

Appendix: Your Hospital Checklists

1. *Twelfth Annual HealthGrades Hospital Quality in America Study.* Golden, CO: HealthGrades Inc., October 2009.

2. Anonymous. "Quaker Tour of England, The Retreat Mental Hospital." Quakerinfo .com. February 12, 2002.

3. Sharon T.A. *Protect Yourself in Hospital.* New York: Contemporary Books, 2004.

Index

About the Authors

Abram Hoffer had a Master's Degree in agricultural chemistry and a Ph.D. in biochemistry. He earned his M.D. from the University of Toronto in 1949 and completed psychiatric residency in 1954. His early work led to the use of niacin for schizophrenia and as an anticholesterol treatment. Dr. Hoffer published over 600 reports and articles as well as 30 books. He died in 2009 at the age of ninety-one.

Andrew W. Saul has over thirty-five years of experience in natural health education, including teaching nutrition, health science, and cell biology at the college level. He is editor of the Orthomolecular Medicine News Service and is featured in the documentary film *FoodMatters*. He is the author of numerous books, including *Doctor Yourself* and *Fire Your Doctor!* (both from Basic Health Publications). His peer-reviewed, non-commercial, natural healing website is DoctorYourself.com.

Steve Hickey has a B.A. (mathematics and science) from the Open University, membership of the Institute of Biology in pharmacology (MI Biol.), and a Ph.D. in medical biophysics from the University of Manchester. He was awarded the Volvo Award for modeling spinal biomechanics, and the Annual Award and Medal of the Back Pain Society. He also researched and developed conformable catheters with Professor John Brocklehurst. He did research into ultra-high-resolution CT scanning and lead the physics team in the clinical MRI unit at Manchester Medical School. More recently, he has been researching cybernetics and decision science at Staffordshire University. He has published over 100 scientific publications and books, and is co-author (with Dr. Saul) of *Vitamin C: The Real Story* (Basic Health Publications).